THE ULTIMATE GUIDE TO INTERMITTENT FASTING FOR WOMEN OVER 50

29 DAYS TO LOSE WEIGHT, FIRE UP YOUR
METABOLISM & DETOX YOUR BODY TO HELP YOU
LOOK AND FEEL YOUR BEST!

FRANCIS HARDING

CONTENTS

INTRODUCTION

One morning, while hurriedly getting ready, I stopped momentarily in front of the mirror. It was one of those rare, unfiltered moments of self-reflection. The face looking back at me had lines I didn't remember and eyes that looked a touch more tired than I felt. "Has it really been that long?" I thought. The memories of younger days, full of energy and vibrancy, seemed distant. "When did I start looking so... aged?" But instead of sinking into that thought, a newfound determination arose. If time wouldn't slow down, I wouldn't let it define me. This was my wake-up call, and I was ready to answer it.

REDISCOVERING OURSELVES: THE SILENT STRUGGLE

At 50, women stand at a unique intersection of life. We've walked paths paved with memories, experienced the ebb and flow of decades, and often reflect on our journey. Yet, as life transitions, so do our bodies, and with it comes waves of different emotions.

Self-confidence, once our second nature, starts to wane as we spot changes in our reflection. Society often paints aging as a decline rather than a shift. More often than not, the narrative pressurizes us to fit into a mold that no longer resonates. The vitality and zest we once felt start to seem like fading memories, replaced by a longing to reclaim the vibrancy that once defined us.

It's not just about vanity; it's about control. It's about wanting to stride confidently into each day, knowing we're at our best. The desire to regain the reins of our health, to feel that familiar surge of energy, becomes more pronounced. And as the world keeps evolving, our yearning to keep pace, to feel our best, and to exude the confidence we once had grows deeper. The journey ahead might seem daunting, but the determination to rediscover ourselves remains undeterred.

DON'T IGNORE THE WAKE-UP CALL

Growing older is about more than just about counting years. For women, it's a dance with change - a dance that's both beautiful and challenging. We see our bodies evolve; sometimes, it feels like we're on a roller coaster without a manual. The wrinkles, the shifts in energy, the unexpected aches - they're all signs of a journey traveled.

Society often ignores us. It's as if, after a certain age, our needs vanish. The beauty and wellness industries? They usually cater to the young, leaving us feeling left out.

But that's where the itch begins. That nagging feeling pushes us to seek answers, to find solutions that fit our unique phase of life. It's not about turning back the clock; it's about feeling great right now. This catalyst - this urge to reclaim our vigor - becomes impossible to ignore.

That's where we come in.

FIVE GAME-CHANGING TAKEAWAYS

At the heart of this book lies a promise: transformation. Intermittent fasting, while beneficial for many, holds unique advantages for women over 50. As you read on, you'll find information made just for you, transforming age-related hurdles into chances for growth. This guide helps you make the most of intermittent fasting, leading to better health, more energy, and renewed confidence in yourself.

- **Made Just for You:** Aging isn't a one-size-fits-all experience. That's why this book is all about you. We've tailored every piece of advice to every strategy, keeping in mind the unique rhythm of a woman's life past 50. No more sifting through generic advice. This is your personalized playbook.
- **No-Guess Meal Plan:** Planning meals can be a chore. But with our 29-day meal plan, you don't need to scratch your head wondering what to eat. We've done the thinking so that you can do the eating. Delicious, nutritious, and designed with variety, keeping you full and completely satisfied.
- **Know Your Metabolism:** Age changes how our bodies work. But instead of just nodding along, let's dive deep. This book helps you understand your metabolism – the why and how of its changes. Knowledge is power, and with this, you'll have the tools to take charge.
- **Detox, the Right Way:** Heard of detoxing but unsure where to begin? We guide you step-by-step. Learn how to cleanse your body, rejuvenate your spirit, and feel the surge of renewed energy. All while ensuring it's safe and effective.

- **A Shoulder to Lean On:** Every journey has its bumps. We know the emotional toll it can sometimes take. This book isn't just a guide but a companion. When things get challenging, as they often do, these pages are here to offer you support, guidance, and encouragement to help you push forward.

Every woman deserves to feel fantastic, no matter her age. With these takeaways, you're not just reading a book but equipping yourself with a healthier, happier journey ahead.

THE SHORTCUTS

Let's be honest: as we gracefully age, we not only earn our stripes in wisdom but also in valuing the beauty of a good shortcut. Why meander the long path when there's a quicker, more efficient route to the goal? The joy of maturity is knowing where to expend energy and where to save it. This book is all about honoring that insight. Here's your ticket to bypassing common Intermittent Fasting pitfalls and diving straight into its rewards. Here's how we help:

- **Straight to the Point:** Dive right in with a clear, step-by-step guide. Kickstart your Intermittent Fasting journey without wading through unnecessary and hard-to-understand jargon or filler.
- **Meal Planning Simplified:** Forget the guesswork. Our 29-day meal plan is here to streamline your meals. It's tailored, efficient, and built to suit your needs, saving you time and effort.
- **Your Concerns Addressed:** Questions? Doubts? We've got you. This guide provides swift and straightforward answers to those common queries that might arise as you navigate your Intermittent Fasting journey.

- **Stay Active, Stay Fit:** Sync your fasting with our fitness advice. Discover exercise tips that are not only aligned with your fasting routine but also customized for your body's unique needs.
- **Social Life, Uninterrupted:** Love socializing? So do I! Get actionable guidance on how to cherish social events and gatherings without swaying from your Intermittent Fasting plan.

STAR POWER: THEY'RE FASTING TOO!

We often picture perfect lives and flawless beauty when we think of celebrities. But guess what? They, too, search for sustainable health practices. With her ageless glow and enviable vitality, Cameron Diaz is a fervent advocate for intermittent fasting. It's not just about Hollywood glam or staying red-carpet-ready; it's about embracing a lifestyle that genuinely enhances health and well-being. Diaz's journey with intermittent fasting reflects its universal appeal. If icons of the screen can trust and benefit from IF, it's a testament to its genuine power in promoting wellness.

A GLIMPSE INTO YOUR VIBRANT TOMORROW

Imagine waking up feeling recharged, not by an alarm clock's rude awakening, but by a natural zest for life. That's just the beginning. By diving deep into intermittent fasting, you're opening the door to a brighter, healthier future.

Your newfound energy isn't a fleeting morning boost. It's here to stay! Whether you're playing with the grandkids, engaging in a spontaneous dance party in your living room, or simply tackling the day's to-do list, you'll notice a massive difference in how you feel. The lethargy that perhaps once held you back?

Gone. Replaced by an unwavering energy that's eager to embrace the day.

Now, let's talk about confidence. We're not just discussing the type that makes you strut a little prouder in your favorite outfit (though there's plenty of that in store!). This is a deeper, unwavering belief in yourself. When you look in the mirror, you'll see a woman who took control, made informed decisions, and reaped the rewards. The reflection staring back? It's one of triumph.

Your mental arena isn't left out. Say goodbye to those foggy moments when names escape you, or you forget tasks. Intermittent fasting brings with it clarity and sharpness. Conversations become more engaging. Books? More immersive. The world just seems a tad brighter.

Socially, you're in for a treat. Confidence and clarity translate to better interactions. You're present, really present, in conversations. Social events become more enjoyable as you navigate them easily, without worrying about food choices or feeling out of place constantly.

Above all, there's a joy, a lightness, and a sense of empowerment. You will realize that you have taken charge of your health and, by extension, your life. The journey through intermittent fasting isn't just about food. It's about rediscovering the joy in every facet of life, from the grand milestones to the everyday moments. Welcome to your vibrant tomorrow.

LIVING PROOF: MY JOURNEY

It's crucial for you to know that I'm not just preaching from a pedestal. I've been where you are. I've felt the insecurities, the challenges, and the weight of age-related changes. My journey with intermittent fasting began years ago, and it wasn't just about research or reading about it. I embraced it wholeheartedly and struggled through its initial challenges, but ultimately, I became stronger and healthier. I've learned, adapted, and transformed throughout the process. The insights I share with you aren't just theoretical; they come from my real-life experiences.

In the following pages, I'll unravel my journey, the peaks and valleys, the victories and the missteps. My aim? To let you learn from my experiences, ensuring you don't trip over the same stones I did. I offer you guidance and advice, not as a distant expert, but as someone who has walked the path, faced its obstacles, and emerged stronger. Consider this book your map, drawn from the terrain of my own journey.

EMBRACING YOUR NEXT CHAPTER

You've made a wise decision in picking up this guide. Out of the many choices available, you've landed on a book crafted specifically for you, the remarkable woman over 50. This book isn't just another generic guide; it's tailored, thoughtful, and resonates with your life's rhythm.

I get it – the hesitations, the need for clarity, the desire for a plan that understands you. And that's precisely what this guide offers. It is a roadmap designed with your unique challenges and aspirations in mind. The upcoming pages aren't just advice but a commitment to your growth, vitality, and rejuvenation.

Feel that flutter in your heart? That's the excitement of transformation, the promise of a vibrant tomorrow. Embrace it. Let's embark on this journey together. Turn the page and ignite the next golden chapter of your life.

1

FOUNDATIONS OF
INTERMITTENT FASTING

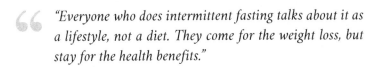 *"Everyone who does intermittent fasting talks about it as a lifestyle, not a diet. They come for the weight loss, but stay for the health benefits."*

— AUTHOR UNKNOWN

As a woman over 50, I've explored many wellness paths, but intermittent fasting truly stood out. I've tried many different approaches to wellness, but intermittent fasting has made a real difference for me. It's more than a passing diet fad; it's proof of how our bodies can flourish and thrive with the proper routine. In this chapter, I'll walk you through the basic ideas, the long-standing history, and the solid science behind intermittent fasting. Together, we'll discover its remarkable benefits for women like us and see that it's more than a health option – it's a life-changing decision.

WHAT IS INTERMITTENT FASTING?

Intermittent fasting, often abbreviated as IF, isn't just about choosing what to eat; it's more about deciding when to eat. It is an eating pattern, a rhythmic cycle of fasting intervals interspersed with periods of unrestricted food intake. Rather than focusing on calorie counting or eliminating certain foods, IF emphasizes the timing of food consumption, allowing the body to experience regular short-term fasts.

When you adopt IF, your body undergoes notable metabolic changes; these changes are rooted in how the body sources its energy. During fasting, instead of relying on glucose from food, the body shifts to using stored fat. This transition not only aids in burning fat but may also benefit heart health, reduce inflammation, and amplify cell repair processes, offering an enhanced metabolic outlook.

Fasting isn't a new-age invention. It's been deeply rooted in various cultures and religious practices for centuries. Early instances of therapeutic intermittent fasts can be traced back to as early as 1915. The 1960s saw a rekindled interest in IF, because of influential reports on its benefits.

Today, intermittent fasting has evolved, tailored to the needs of diverse demographics, including vibrant women over 50 like us! Recognizing the unique metabolic and hormonal changes women experience in this age group, modern IF techniques have been adapted to suit these needs. Studies suggest that for women in this stage, IF can bring similar benefits as continuous energy restriction but may come with added advantages like reduced hunger and improved adherence.

Various schedules or patterns have emerged over the years. While the foundation remains the same—alternate between eating and fasting periods—the duration and frequency can vary. Martin Berkhan, credited as an inventor of a popular IF method, paved the way in 2006. Whether it's the 16/8 method, where you fast for 16 hours and eat during an 8-hour window or alternate-day fasting, each pattern offers a unique approach to fit individual lifestyles and goals.

THE SCIENCE BEHIND IF

At its core, IF revolves around the principle of cycling between eating and fasting periods by focusing more on when you eat rather than what you eat. During fasting, your body undergoes a series of metabolic changes, tapping into stored fat for energy, which can lead to weight loss. Additionally, IF can prompt cellular repair processes in the body, reducing inflammation and providing significant benefits for heart-health. The beauty of IF is that it mirrors ancient human eating patterns, aligning with periods when food was abundant and when it wasn't.

Human Metabolism 101:

Think of metabolism as your body's engine. It's the process of converting what you eat and drink into energy. Even at rest, our bodies need energy for breathing, circulating blood, and cell repair. This energy is measured in calories. The rate at which our body uses these calories is termed metabolic rate. Various factors, like age, muscle mass, and activity levels, affect it. When you eat, your metabolism speeds up to digest food.

On the other hand, fasting provides energy to the body by burning fat. It must alter the body's metabolic process and rate and begin breaking down fat stores to use for fuel. Understanding this helps in grasping the potential of IF.

Starvation State vs. Fasting:

Many mistakenly believe that fasting and starving are the same, but they're fundamentally different. Let's clear up the confusion.

Fasting is a deliberate, controlled, and temporary absence from food, often with a specific goal in mind – be it for health, spiritual, or other reasons. When we fast, our body taps into stored energy (like fat) for fuel after its primary energy source, glucose, runs low. This process is a natural response and can offer numerous benefits, such as improved metabolic health and cellular repair. Most importantly, we choose when to start and end a fast.

Starvation, however, is a prolonged lack of essential nutrients the body needs to function correctly. It's involuntary. Starvation isn't about tapping into fat reserves for a day or so; it's when the body has depleted its fat and starts breaking down vital tissues, like muscles, for energy. This state can lead to severe health complications driven by necessity, not choice.

In essence, fasting is a strategic pause in food intake, giving our bodies a break. At the same time, starvation is a forced, harmful deprivation. Knowing this distinction ensures we approach IF safely and effectively, maximizing benefits without harming our health.

Balancing the Scales: The Pros and Cons of Intermittent Fasting

Introducing a new approach to eating, especially one as transformative as Intermittent Fasting (IF), requires a holistic view. So, while the advocates swear by its many benefits, it's only fair to shed light on its potential downsides. Let's take an informed dive into both sides of the IF coin.

✚ Pros:

- **Weight Management:** IF has been praised for its effectiveness in weight loss. By eating during specific windows, our body learns to burn stored fat for energy.
- **Improved Metabolic Health:** Studies suggest that IF can enhance insulin sensitivity, thus reducing the risk of type 2 diabetes.
- **Heart Health:** Intermittent fasting may lead to beneficial changes in blood pressure, cholesterol levels, triglycerides, and inflammatory markers.
- **Cellular Repair and Longevity:** Fasting triggers autophagy, where cells remove faulty parts, potentially prolonging efficient functioning.
- **Brain Health:** IF boosts the production of a brain-derived neurotrophic factor (BDNF) hormone, enhancing brain function and reducing the risk of neurodegenerative diseases.

▬ Cons:

- **Hunger and Fatigue:** Initially, you might experience hunger pangs and fatigue, which can be challenging to push through.
- **Overeating in Eating Windows:** There's a temptation to overindulge during eating periods, which might counteract the benefits of fasting.
- **Potential Nutrient Deficiency:** With careful planning, you might get essential nutrients.
- **Social and Lifestyle Impact:** Fasting might clash with social outings or family meals.
- **Might Not Suit Everyone:** Certain individuals, especially those with specific health issues or those pregnant, are advised against IF.

Intermittent fasting can be a helpful tool for health and weight, but it's not one-size-fits-all. Remember, everyone's journey is unique. If you face challenges with intermittent fasting, don't worry. This guide has plenty of advice and solutions to address those issues, helping you find a routine that fits your lifestyle and goals. Remember that before you start, it's a good idea to chat with a doctor.

Shedding Pounds with Intermittent Fasting

Intermittent Fasting (IF) has risen in popularity not just as a fad but because of its authentic, science-backed benefits for weight management. Let's dive into the mechanisms of how IF assists in weight reduction.

Insulin Levels: One of the core principles of IF revolves around insulin. This hormone stores sugar in the liver and prompts the body to store fat. When fasting, insulin levels drop significantly, allowing the body to release stored sugar and burn stored fat for energy.

Boosted Metabolism: Research has shown that short-term fasting can increase metabolic rate by 3.6% to 14%, helping your body burn even more calories. A boosted metabolism means, during an IF regime, not only are you potentially eating less, but your body is burning calories at a faster pace.

Norepinephrine Production: Fasting stimulates the production of norepinephrine, a neurotransmitter that boosts metabolism. When norepinephrine communicates with fat cells, it breaks them down into free fatty acids, which the body burns for energy.

Mindful Eating: Limiting the eating window encourages better food choices. While this is more of a behavioral change than a biological one, it's essential to why many people succeed with IF.

Hormonal Advantage: Apart from insulin, IF impacts several other hormones like the hunger hormone ghrelin and the fullness hormone leptin. These advantages can lead to reduced appetite and make weight loss more manageable.

Intermittent Fasting is more than just an eating pattern—it's a science-backed approach that optimizes your body's hormonal and metabolic functions to favor weight loss. IF can be a potent ally when adopted mindfully in your weight management journey.

Continuous Calorie Restriction vs. Intermittent Fasting

Two leading strategies emerge at the heart of most weight loss discussions: Continuous Calorie Restriction (CCR) and Intermittent Fasting (IF). Both approaches have their merits, but how do they compare against each other?

Continuous Calorie Restriction (CCR) is anchored in a straight-forward concept. By consistently reducing daily caloric intake, often by 20% to 40%, you aim to consume fewer calories than your body expends. Over time, this should naturally result in weight loss. While simple and direct, the approach offers steady results for those who adhere to it strictly. However, its continuous nature can make it challenging to sustain in the long run. Additionally, if not paired with a well-balanced diet, it can lead to muscle loss and may gradually slow down metabolism. The nutrients we get from our foods feed our cells, support body functions, and help repair and grow new tissues, keeping us energetic and healthy as we age.

On the other side of the spectrum, Intermittent Fasting (IF) shifts the focus. Instead of concentrating on how much you eat, the emphasis is on when you eat. Typically, this method involves cycles of eating and fasting, such as the popular 16-hour fast followed by an 8-hour eating window. The beauty of IF is that it often leads to automatic calorie restriction without the need for meticulous counting. Short-term fasts can even give the metabolism a boost while also positively influencing several weight-loss hormones. However, transitioning into IF can come with challenges like initial hunger pangs. And, like CCR, it might not be a one-size-fits-all solution, especially for individuals with certain medical conditions.

Both strategies have their unique merits. Throughout the years, I tried many different diets, searching for the one that would fit into my lifestyle and help me feel my best. I recall the period I tried CCR, diligently tracking every calorie and ensuring I stayed within my daily limit. While I noticed some changes, the constant counting became mentally taxing. That's when I stumbled upon Intermittent Fasting. The freedom from counting calories, paired with the structured eating windows, truly resonated with me. It felt less restrictive and more in tune with my body's natural rhythms. Plus, the noticeable improvements in my energy levels and overall well-being sealed the deal. Of course, everyone's journey is personal. What worked for me might not work for you. So, as you contemplate which path to choose, consider your lifestyle, preferences, and unique health circumstances.

UNIQUE BENEFITS OF IF FOR WOMEN OVER 50

Navigating the golden years gracefully involves understanding the distinct challenges and possibilities. Especially for women over 50, this phase is a blend of transformation and rediscovery. While the journey is unique for each of us, certain universal truths ring true. Our body undergoes significant hormonal, metabolic, and emotional changes as we age. The good news? Intermittent Fasting (IF) offers a suite of benefits tailored to address these very shifts. Whether you want to manage menopausal symptoms, boost metabolism, or achieve sustainable weight loss, IF might be the ticket.

Managing Hormonal Changes

The golden years after 50 often come with a suite of changes, particularly those related to hormones. Menopause, that inevitable phase for every woman, brings a flurry of symptoms like hot flashes, mood swings, and sometimes sleep disturbances. Now, imagine if there was a way to ease this natural transition.

Research suggests that IF can potentially alleviate some menopausal symptoms. By aligning our eating patterns with our circadian rhythms, IF might play a role in stabilizing hormone fluctuations, notably insulin levels. Improved insulin sensitivity could pave the way for better sleep and mood stabilization.

On a personal note, I recall those nights when hot flashes would rudely interrupt my dreams, leaving me flustered and craving solace. When I started on my IF journey, it wasn't just about weight loss. To my astonishment, within weeks, my sleep improved, and the intensity of hot flashes diminished. While every woman's journey through menopause is unique, the promise of potential relief made IF an appealing choice for me. Whether you're exploring IF for similar reasons or others, it's worth noting that, as with any approach, individual experiences may vary. But sometimes, amidst the turbulence of menopause, even a little relief can feel like a gentle, welcoming breeze.

The IF Weight Loss Advantage

Weight loss often feels like an uphill battle, particularly after reaching 50. With metabolic rates naturally slowing down and hormonal fluctuations playing their part, shedding those extra pounds might seem more challenging than before. But here's where Intermittent Fasting (IF) offers a glimmer of hope.

One of the primary reasons intermittent fasting (IF) may be particularly effective for you is that it can improve insulin sensitivity. Intermittent fasting helps improve how your body uses insulin. As we get older, our body sometimes struggles to use insulin properly, which can cause weight gain. With IF, there are times when your insulin levels are lower. Because of this, your body burns fat and uses stored fat for energy more efficiently.

Moreover, IF can bring about a sense of discipline in your eating habits. Being more mindful about what you eat can naturally lead to reduced calorie intake, making weight loss more attainable.

Lastly, there's a mental aspect. Reaching 50 is an achievement, and with it comes maturity and determination. Embracing IF at this stage means you're likely approaching it with commitment, understanding its nuances, and harnessing its benefits for a fitter you. It's not just a dietary shift; it's a lifestyle choice that can be a game-changer for many women in this golden phase.

The Cognitive Edge of IF

For many, the golden years represent a time of reflection, joy, and the culmination of life's experiences. Yet, an undercurrent of concern often shadows this phase: the potential for cognitive decline. This apprehension is particularly valid for women, as they statistically bear a higher risk for conditions like Alzheimer's disease. But what if a simple dietary pattern could buffer against this decline?

Enter Intermittent Fasting (IF), not just as a weight loss technique but as a formidable ally for brain health. One of the most promising revelations from IF research is its capacity to elevate levels of a vital protein called brain-derived neurotrophic factor (BDNF). Think of BDNF as a kind of 'fertilizer' for the brain—it nurtures neural pathways, fosters the birth of new neurons, and fortifies existing ones.

Enhanced BDNF levels, catalyzed by IF, are linked to improved memory, sharper focus, and heightened cognitive agility. More than just offering a transient boost, elevated BDNF can present a formidable defense against neurodegenerative diseases. For women over 50, adopting an IF regimen can be a strategic move, not just for the body but for the mind. It's a proactive step towards ensuring their later years are golden and vibrant.

IF to Boost Bone Health

As we journey through life, we must face many ups and downs. As women gracefully transition past menopause, they face a quiet yet significant challenge – the natural decrease in bone density. If unchecked, this subtle thinning of bones can lead to conditions like osteoporosis, making them more susceptible to fractures from even minor falls. It's a concern that holds many women back, keeping them from participating in activities they love for fear of being injured.

However, there's an emerging beacon of hope in Intermittent Fasting (IF). Beyond its known benefits for weight loss and metabolic health, IF reveals its prowess in an unexpected domain – bone health. How does it achieve this? By amplifying the body's natural ability to absorb calcium, the primary building block for bones. Adequate calcium uptake ensures bones remain robust, dense, and resilient against potential fractures.

Furthermore, studies have suggested that IF can encourage the production of osteoblasts – the specialized cells responsible for new bone growth. These cells not only aid in repairing minor damages but also ensure continued bone strength.

As you get older, incorporating IF into your lifestyle isn't just about losing weight; it's also about strengthening your bones and enhancing your body's foundation. A foundation that ensures every step taken is on robust and unwavering ground, allowing you to stride forward with confidence and grace.

The Skin-Reviving Power of IF

With the golden years comes the rich tapestry of experiences that paint stories on our faces. These stories manifest as wrinkles, fine lines, and other subtle changes that the skin undergoes, shaped by time and hormonal shifts. While these changes are a testament to the journey traveled, they also spark a longing to retain that youthful radiance and suppleness.

That's where intermittent fasting comes in. It's not just a transformative tool for weight or metabolism but a potent ally for your skin. How? At the heart of IF's skin-enhancing magic lies a remarkable process called autophagy. Think of autophagy as nature's spa treatment, a 'clean-up' mechanism where the body meticulously removes worn-out, damaged cells, making room for fresh, vibrant ones.

When embracing IF, you effectively cue your body to initiate this rejuvenation process more frequently. The result? A visible reduction in age spots, fine lines, and wrinkles gives way to skin that's not only more elastic and firm but also radiates a youthful glow.

So, IF offers a promising path for those seeking a natural way to rekindle that inner and outer glow. It's not just about looking younger; it's about feeling invigorated, knowing that a meticulous process is continually working to unveil your most radiant self beneath the surface.

DECODING THE METABOLIC MAGIC: IF'S INFLUENCE ON WEIGHT AND WELLNESS

Navigating the golden years of my life, I vividly recall my frustration with the seemingly relentless weight gain. The scales didn't reflect the energetic, youthful spirit I felt inside. Even more perplexing was my slowing metabolism, a common complaint I'd hear from my peers over our weekly brunches. That's when I stumbled upon Intermittent Fasting (IF) and the growing body of research supporting its role in metabolic recalibration and weight loss.

Empirical Studies: Validating IF's Efficacy for Women Over 50

Science shows intermittent fasting has many benefits, especially for women over 50. Studies have found that IF can help people with obesity lose weight and have better overall health. It's not just a trendy fad; fundamental research is behind it to back it up.

Also, specific studies show that IF can benefit women after menopause. As hormone levels fluctuate and the body undergoes myriad changes, IF emerges as a potential stabilizer, harmonizing these shifts. It's worth noting that while the internet is awash with claims about IF's ability to rev up metabolism, it's essential to discern fact from fiction. Most credible research suggests that Intermittent Fasting doesn't merely prevent a metabolic slowdown (a common concern with many dieting strategies) but might also amplify fat-burning hormones, further solidifying its role as a powerful weight management tool.

The Art and Science of Shedding Pounds with IF

When you embark on the Intermittent Fasting journey, it's like setting the stage for a metabolic ballet inside your body. Here's how it works: Typically after you eat, your body works on digesting and absorbing that food. During this time, insulin levels are high, making fat-burning challenging. As time progresses and you don't eat (like when you're fasting), insulin levels drop. Lower insulin levels send a green light for your body to start burning stored fat for energy.

Furthermore, IF enhances the release of norepinephrine, a fat-burning hormone. This hormonal duo—lowered insulin and increased norepinephrine—amplifies the body's fat-burning potential. Additionally, by cycling between eating and fasting, you naturally consume fewer calories, promoting weight loss. It's an elegant dance of hormones and energy, aligning perfectly to help you achieve a healthier you.

At its core, IF introduces periods of little to no caloric intake. During these fasting windows, some remarkable things start happening at the cellular level:

- **Cellular Autophagy:** One of the standout benefits of IF is its ability to stimulate autophagy, a process where cells dispose of damaged components, making room for newer, more efficient parts. Think of it as the body's recycling system. This enhanced cellular 'clean-up' ensures that metabolic processes run smoother and more efficiently.

- **Optimized Insulin Sensitivity:** Insulin plays a pivotal role in regulating blood sugar levels. With age, insulin resistance can develop, where cells no longer respond to insulin as they should. This slowdown can lead to weight gain and energy lags. Intermittent fasting promotes lower insulin levels during fasting periods, allowing the body to improve its sensitivity to the hormone. As a result, cells become better equipped to uptake glucose, driving more consistent energy levels and supporting metabolic health.

- **Enhanced Fat Oxidation:** During prolonged fasting windows, when the readily available glucose runs low, the body turns to its fat reserves for energy. This process, termed fat oxidation, becomes more predominant, helping to break down and utilize stored fat effectively.

- **Hormonal Synergy:** IF also plays a role in fine-tuning various hormones that influence metabolism. Besides insulin, hormones like norepinephrine see an uptick during fasting. This hormone aids in mobilizing fat cells to be converted into energy.

The science behind IF's ability to boost metabolism revolves around harnessing the body's natural processes, amplifying them, and creating an environment where metabolic functions are rejuvenated. By providing the body with strategic breaks from constant digestion and caloric intake, IF allows it to 'reset', reinvigorate, and re-engage with its metabolic duties, leading to a more vibrant, energized you.

DEBUNKING IF MYTHS AND SETTING THE RECORD STRAIGHT

Navigating the world of Intermittent Fasting can sometimes feel like traversing a maze. With so much information available, it's easy to stumble upon misconceptions, half-truths, and outright myths. As someone who's adopted IF as part of my journey, I've encountered countless queries, concerns, and misunderstandings from friends, colleagues, and even my initial beliefs. In this section, we'll uncover some common misconceptions about intermittent fasting. We will use real research to separate fact from fiction to ensure you start your journey with clarity. Doing so will educate you about IF and give you the confidence you need to start your journey with a solid first step.

- **Intermittent Fasting is Best for Weight Loss:** While IF can be a successful weight loss strategy for many, it's not necessarily the "best" for everyone. Weight loss success varies with personal preferences, lifestyle, and metabolic responses. Remember, the most effective diet is the one you can maintain.
- **You Can't Get Enough Nutrients if You Fast:** A shorter eating window doesn't mean nutrient deficiency. It's about quality, not quantity. You can still meet your nutritional needs by focusing on nutrient-dense foods during your eating periods. That's one of the great things about our 29-day meal plan. It ensures you get all the nutrient-rich food your body requires to function at its absolute best.
- **You Can't Exercise When You're Fasting:** Exercising during a fast is entirely possible. Some even feel more endurance and focus. It's essential, however, to listen to your body. If you're feeling weak, consider adjusting your workout intensity or timing.

- **Fasting Will Extend Your Life:** The research on fasting and lifespan extension is still emerging. While some animal studies show promise, we can't conclusively state that fasting guarantees a longer life in humans. We know that IF can improve markers of health, which might contribute to longevity.

- **You'll Lose Muscle if You're Doing Intermittent Fasting:** While it's essential to maintain protein intake, IF doesn't inherently cause muscle loss; ensuring adequate protein and incorporating resistance training can help maintain muscle mass during IF. Our 29-day meal plan includes plenty of foods with sufficient amounts of protein to ensure that your body stays strong and your muscles have the chance to grow. You won't feel weak, tired, or hungry, and trust me, your muscles will thank you for it.

- **Skipping Breakfast is Unhealthy:** Breakfast's importance varies by individual. For some, skipping breakfast and eating later can be beneficial, while others thrive with a morning meal. It's about tuning into your body's needs.

- **IF is the Miracle Cure for Weight Loss:** Intermittent fasting can be an excellent tool for many, but it's not a magic fix that works the same for everyone. Your success with it will be shaped by consistency, the types of foods you choose during eating windows, and your personal health and daily routines. It's all about finding the right balance that suits your individual needs.

- **All Intermittent Fasting is the Same:** There are several IF variations, from 16/8 and 5:2 to alternate-day fasting. Each has nuances and potential benefits, so finding a pattern that aligns with your lifestyle and health goals is crucial.

- **IF is Good for Everyone:** Intermittent fasting offers benefits, but it's not universal. Some people, particularly those with certain medical conditions or women who are pregnant, may not find it suitable. It's essential to consult a healthcare professional before starting.
- **IF Can Impair Your Mental Alertness and Focus:** While some experience clarity during fasting, others might face temporary fog. This hurdle usually passes as the body adjusts to using fat as fuel.
- **Intermittent Fasting Slows Down Your Metabolism:** On the contrary, short-term fasting might boost your metabolism by stimulating norepinephrine production. Prolonged calorie restriction, not intermittent fasting, can decrease metabolic rate.
- **Intermittent Fasting Makes You Overindulge:** While some fear they'd binge post-fasting, practicing mindful eating can prevent this. The body learns to crave what it genuinely needs, guiding you towards more balanced choices.
- **You Are Supposed to Restrict Your Water Intake During the Fasting Window:** Many fall prey to this false belief. Hydration is essential, regardless of fasting. During your fasting window, drinking water, herbal teas, or black coffee is encouraged to maintain hydration and support the body's natural detoxification processes.
- **Intermittent Fasting Puts Your Body into Starvation Mode:** Intermittent fasting is different from prolonged starvation. Short-term fasting can increase metabolism, whereas continuous, very low-calorie intake may trigger a decrease in metabolic rate.
- **You Can't Gain Muscle While Fasting:** Not true. Muscle growth is possible during intermittent fasting

with appropriate strength training and protein intake during eating windows.

- **Fasting Saps Your Energy:** Some people experience a surge in energy due to increased norepinephrine production during fasting. While adjusting might take time, many report heightened alertness and energy once they acclimate to the fasting routine.

Diving into the world of health and nutrition, you'll bump into myths left and right – especially when something like intermittent fasting takes the spotlight. As we've seen, it's clear that a lot of what's "common knowledge" about IF might be a half-truth or a misunderstood snippet. So, when considering trying out a trend or making any significant change, always take a step back, chat with professionals, or even trust your gut. Your path to well-being is your unique adventure, and it's all about finding what truly clicks for you amidst all the chatter.

CHECKLIST FOR SUCCESS: MASTERING INTERMITTENT FASTING

- **DIY Your IF Style:** There's no one-size-fits-all approach to IF. Whether you gravitate towards a 16/8 regimen or the 5:2 method, tailor your fasting to what feels suitable for you. We will explore all of the different fasting methods in detail later on.
- **Consult With Your Doctor:** Before starting your IF journey, it's always wise to check in with your healthcare professional. An informed start is a smart start.
- **Stay Hydrated:** Water is your trusty sidekick in this adventure. It'll help quell those hunger pangs and keep you feeling refreshed.

- **Breaking the Fast with Finesse:** When it's time to refuel, opt for nutrient-rich choices. Later on, you can have a more substantial meal without any guilt.
- **Prioritize Sleep:** Good rest goes hand in hand with good health. Make sure to catch those Z's for a refreshed you.
- **Gather Your Support Crew:** Encourage friends or family to join the IF bandwagon. Sharing experiences and tips can make the journey smoother and more enjoyable.
- **Moderation is Key:** While IF provides more flexibility, maintaining balance is essential. Overindulging after fasting can counteract the benefits.
- **Celebrate the Benefits:** From enhancing brain health to improving metabolism, always remember the myriad benefits of IF. It serves as excellent motivation.
- **Mindful Eating:** Relish every bite. Take the time to savor your meals, understanding the nourishment they provide.
- **Beyond Just a Diet:** Remember, IF isn't merely a diet; it's a lifestyle shift. It's not strictly about the foods you consume but also the timing.

Help! I'm Hungry

→ **Stay Hydrated:** Drinking plenty of water can make you feel full for longer. Plus, it keeps your body well-hydrated.

→ **Herbal Teas:** Warm, calming, and a great distraction. Herbal teas can provide a soothing ritual without adding calories.

→ **Distraction Techniques:** Dive into a hobby, immerse yourself in a book, or go for a short walk. Sometimes, the mind needs a brief diversion.

→ **Bubble It Up:** Sparkling water can feel more filling than its still counterpart. The fizz can be quite satisfying!

→ **Mindful Breathing:** A quick meditation or deep breathing exercise can help center you, taking your focus off the hunger.

→ **Chew on This:** While you shouldn't make a habit of it, chewing gum can occasionally act as a stop-gap till your next meal.

→ **Know Your Body:** Remember, there's a difference between true hunger and mere boredom or thirst. Learning to differentiate can be invaluable.

Breaking Your Fast: Do It Right

★ **Slow and Steady:** Start with something light, like a handful of nuts or a piece of fruit, to gently introduce food back into your system.

★ **Hydrate First:** Before eating, have a glass of water. Hydration can prepare your stomach and help you feel fuller more quickly.

★ **Lean on Protein:** Protein-rich foods like lean meats or legumes can be satiating and provide the energy boost you're likely craving.

★ **Mind the Fiber:** Incorporate fiber-rich foods like vegetables. They help with digestion and offer a slow, steady source of energy.

★ **Avoid Overloading on Sugars:** It might be tempting to reach for something sweet, but this can cause a rapid spike and crash in blood sugar. Stick to natural sugars like fruits if you need something sweet.

★ **Listen to Your Body:** Pay attention to how different foods make you feel when breaking your fast. Over time, you'll recognize what best suits your body.

Tying It All Together

Wow, time flies when you dive deep into something as transformative as intermittent fasting, right? In this chapter, we've come a long way, piecing together the IF mosaic, especially for women over 50. We've laid a sturdy groundwork from busting those pesky myths to giving you the low-down on managing those "I'm so hungry!" moments.

But here's a little secret: before we really immerse ourselves in the world of fasting, we have more prep work. Think of it as the warm-up before a good workout. Our next step is all about detoxification. No, it's not just about those fancy green smoothies or luxe spa days (though they sound lovely!). It's about getting our bodies and minds in tip-top shape to fully embrace the benefits of fasting.

So, are you ready to roll up your sleeves and dive into the rejuvenating realm of detox? Let's make our next chapter all about that perfect prep!

2

DETOXIFYING YOUR BODY

"You can enhance your body's natural detoxification system by simply changing your diet."

— UNKNOWN AUTHOR

Back in the day, after one too many holiday treats or indulgent weekends, I'd often tell my friends, "I just wish there was a reset button for my body!" Little did I know that our bodies, in their intricate wisdom, have designed one all along: the art of detoxification. When I started learning more about health and wellness, I discovered how closely detox and intermittent fasting connect. In this chapter, we'll explore the process of our body's natural cleansing system. I'll share personal stories about my own experiences and the unique facts about our body's ability to refresh and rejuvenate.

WHAT IS DETOX?

Detoxification, commonly known as detox, is the body's natural, ongoing process of neutralizing and eliminating toxins. These toxins can be external (environmental chemicals, pesticides in food, alcohol, or drugs) and internal (waste products from regular cellular activity). The body has its dedicated 'clean-up crew,' mainly the liver, kidneys, lungs, skin, and lymphatic system, tirelessly working to filter and expel these undesirables.

But let's break it down a bit. Imagine your body as a bustling city. Over time, waste accumulates. If left unchecked, this waste can hinder the city's function. That's where the detox process enters. It acts as the sanitation department, ensuring the city remains clean and operates at its peak.

However, in today's world, we often find ourselves exposed to an increasing number of harmful substances. From processed foods to pollution, these toxins can strain our natural detox system, just like how even the most efficient city cleaning crew might need help after a major event or storm.

This is where the idea of intentional detoxing comes in. Individuals can support and boost their body's natural detoxification process through specific diets, supplements, therapies, or practices. The goal? To rid the body of accumulated toxins, refresh the system, and thereby improve overall health and vitality.

Knowing this, the power of detox becomes clearer. It's not just about cleansing; it's about rejuvenating and empowering your body to function at its best.

Autophagy: Nature's Cleaning Crew

You know that exhilarating feeling after you've decluttered your closet, getting rid of old clothes and making space for the new? Your body has its version of spring cleaning, and it's called autophagy. Trust us; it's even more fantastic than finding that shirt you thought you'd lost forever.

Autophagy, derived from the Greek words for "self-eating," is your body's way of tidying up. When activated, cells go into survival mode, breaking down and recycling their worn-out parts. It's like your body's internal recycling program, ensuring everything runs efficiently and no unnecessary junk piles up.

So, why should you be excited about this cellular housekeeping?

- **Cellular Health:** At its core, autophagy breaks down cell components that are damaged or no longer useful. This recycling of cellular material aids in cell renewal, ensuring the optimal performance of each cell. In simpler terms? It's like replacing old, worn-out machinery with newer, efficient models.
- **Brain Health:** There's compelling research to suggest that autophagy supports cognitive function. Decluttering the cellular debris in neural pathways potentially reduces the risk of neurodegenerative diseases. Think of it as your brain's personal maintenance crew, ensuring the pathways are clear and connections swift.
- **Boosted Immunity:** Autophagy indirectly strengthens the immune system by promoting the disposal of old, damaged cellular components. This process ensures you're better equipped to fight off those pesky pathogens. Imagine bolstering your castle's walls against invaders; that's autophagy for your immune system.

- **Enhanced Metabolism:** Enhanced autophagy can lead to improved metabolic responses. Promoting efficient cellular operations aids in better insulin sensitivity and robust fat metabolism. Picture it as your body's engine getting a tune-up for peak performance.

Now, let's tie this into intermittent fasting (IF). IF serves as a catalyst for autophagy. When you fast, you signal your cells to start this self-cleaning process. So, while you're aiming for weight loss or better metabolic health with IF, your cells are reaping the rewards of autophagy.

The Benefits of Detox

When I first dabbled in the wellness world, "detox" was a term I'd often encounter, accompanied by all sorts of mixed feelings. Some thought it was just a passing trend, others saw it as a transformative process. I was curious and wanted to learn more, so I started looking into detox. I realized that detoxification wasn't just a periodic cleanse but a journey toward optimal well-being. There's so much I learned from this, both physically and mentally. Let me share the incredible revelations I learned about detox and how it can significantly impact your health journey.

- **Natural Purification:** Early in my wellness journey, I understood detox as a profound cleanse, akin to spring cleaning for our bodies. Through detox, we actively support our bodies in eliminating toxins, creating a renewed vibrancy. Imagine walking into a decluttered and freshly aired room - there's an invigorating clarity, right? That's what detox can do for your insides.
- **Optimal Functionality:** The more I learned about detox, the more I noticed how it can significantly affect

how our bodies function. When toxins don't bog down our systems, they perform as nature intended. This translates to improved digestion, increased ability to absorb nutrients, and a notable enhancement in several other bodily functions. It's like tuning up a car; once you've changed the oil and checked all the parts, it runs with a purr.

- **A Boosted Mood:** One of the most delightful surprises in my detox journey was the uplifting change in my emotional landscape. As our bodies shed waste, there's a palpable lift in energy and emotional equilibrium. You know that gentle euphoria after a deep, restful meditation? Detox, in many ways, replicates that feeling at a cellular level.

- **Enhanced Immunity:** As I became more attuned to my body post-detox, I noticed fewer sniffles and aches. With fewer toxins acting as hurdles, our immune system finds its rhythm, efficiently guarding against illnesses. Picture an athlete on a cleared track, every stride stronger without obstructions. That's your immune system thriving post-detox.

THE CONNECTION BETWEEN IF AND DETOX

When I began my wellness journey, intermittent fasting (IF) and detoxification initially seemed like two separate paths. But, as I delved deeper, a revelation dawned: they were interconnected, complementing each other like two sides of the same coin. IF isn't merely a dietary approach; it's a bridge that connects us to our body's innate healing and detoxifying capabilities—the profound effects of fasting stretch beyond the commonly recognized weight loss benefits. From rejuvenating our brain and gut to enhancing our heart's health, the interplay of IF and detox is truly astounding. In this section, let's explore this symbiotic relationship and understand the intricate dance between fasting and our body's detoxification process. Whether you're an IF enthusiast or just beginning to dip your toes into its waters, this section will provide a holistic understanding of its rejuvenating powers.

The Synergistic Relationship Between IF and Detox

Science has revealed to us the hidden ways our body works. When it comes to detoxification, the body has its built-in mechanisms. Adding intermittent fasting into your routine can enhance these detox methods and make them even better.

A study conducted in the Cell Stem Cell journal found that cycles of prolonged fasting, which are principles at the heart of IF, activate stem cell regeneration of new immune cells, effectively renewing the immune system. This reinvigoration allows for a more robust response to toxins and pathogens.

Now, consider the liver, our primary detox organ. It works diligently to neutralize unwanted toxins from our diet or environment. During periods of fasting, our insulin levels drop, which promotes lipolysis, the breakdown of fat cells. This process metabolizes and excretes toxins stored in fat deposits, cleaning our internal environment.

Moreover, a fascinating phenomenon comes into play: autophagy. Without external food sources during fasting, our cells begin a process where they "eat" and break down malfunctioning or unused components, thereby detoxifying at a cellular level. According to a 2016 Nature Reviews Molecular Cell Biology report, this isn't just about cleaning house; it positively impacts cellular efficiency and longevity.

Lastly, consider the gut. Balancing the gut microbiome can promote a favorable gut environment through IF. A balanced gut means better detoxification, with fewer harmful bacteria producing endotoxins.

In a nutshell, IF doesn't just intersect with detox; it amplifies it. The science confirms it: fasting provides the body with the optimum environment to naturally cleanse and rejuvenate. It's not just a dietary pattern; it's a strategic approach for holistic well-being.

Science Behind IF-Induced Autophagy

Let's demystify the word "autophagy" first. It might sound complex, but its essence is relatively straightforward. As we mentioned earlier, the term comes from the Greek words "auto" (self) and "phagein" (to eat). So, autophagy literally means "self-eating". Now, before you conjure up some bizarre mental image, let's unpack this fascinating concept.

Our bodies, like every well-oiled machine, sometimes need to undergo maintenance. Autophagy is one such maintenance process. It's where our cells tidy up by removing damaged parts, ensuring everything runs smoothly. Think of it as your body's housekeeping service.

How does intermittent fasting (IF) trigger this? When you fast, nutrient levels in your cells drop. This drop is a signal for the body to start conserving energy. Instead of generating new parts, cells start recycling old ones, triggering autophagy.

According to research published in the journal Nature Communications, this isn't just about cleaning up; it's about survival. Autophagy prevents damaged proteins and cells from accumulating, which can lead to diseases. It's like ensuring you regularly service your car to avoid major breakdowns.

To put it simply, by practicing IF, you're not just losing weight or achieving metabolic benefits. You're also giving your cells the much-needed opportunity to clean, repair, and rejuvenate. It's nature's way of ensuring you keep running in tip-top shape.

Key Considerations for Detox

Are you embarking on a detox journey? It's not just about skipping meals or resisting that tempting chocolate chip cookie. Fasting, particularly for detoxification, is more nuanced than it might first appear. While the modern world has just discovered the wonders of fasting, our ancestors intuitively understood its potential benefits. From improving insulin sensitivity to reducing the risk of chronic diseases, fasting is more than just a dietary whim – it's a strategic move toward optimal health.

However, stepping into this realm with both eyes open is essential. While Angus Barbieri's record-breaking 382-day fast might leave you awe-inspired; remember, detoxification and fasting are deeply personal journeys. What works for one might not suit another. Not every fasting regimen is exclusively about "detoxification"; some are researched for their potential in health promotion, disease prevention, and weight loss.

But before you set your detox timer, know this: genuine detoxification kicks in after about 12 hours of fasting. It's that magical phase where the body gets down to the business of internal housekeeping. And as you wade through the waters of fasting, remember to keep hydrated. Water isn't just about quenching thirst; it's the body's primary detox agent, regulating temperature, aiding digestion, and flushing out toxins. Other nutrient-rich drinks are also a game-changer when you detox. Drinks high in electrolytes (such as the Liquid IV drink packets) can rehydrate your body and provide it with everything necessary to boost detoxification.

Dive in with awareness, arm yourself with the proper knowledge, and respect the unique rhythm of your body. After all, detoxification isn't a race; it's a journey toward a healthier, revitalized you.

How to Detoxify Successfully and Stay Nourished

When you first hear about fasting, you might picture an empty plate and a rumbling stomach. But let's shift that image a little. Think of fasting not as deprivation but rather as a vacation for your digestive system, a reset button for your body, and a detox boost. Now, doesn't that sound more appealing?

- **Start Gradually:** Instead of plunging into a prolonged fast, why not dip your toes in first? Begin with shorter intervals, maybe 8 or 10 hours, and as your body acclimates, extend the duration. Your body will thank you for this gentle introduction.
- **Hydration is Key:** Water should be your steadfast companion while your food intake is on a mini-break. It's the silent hero that aids in flushing out toxins, keeping your cells hydrated, and maintaining your energy levels.
- **Listen to Your Body:** This can't be stressed enough. If you're feeling off, excessively tired, or just not right – it might be a cue to modify your approach. Remember, it's about wellness, not endurance.
- **Nourish Between Fasts:** When you do eat, make it count. Focus on whole, nutritious foods packed with vitamins and minerals. Healthy eating isn't just about detoxifying but rejuvenating and nourishing your body post-fast.

Fasting Detox: Foods & Drinks

Remember, just because you're taking a break from eating during specific periods doesn't mean you can't be mindful of what you consume when it's time to break your fast. Here's a curated list to guide you on foods and drinks that can amplify the detox effects of fasting:

- **Water, Water, Water!:** While fasting, hydration should be your mantra. The more water you drink, the better you will feel and the more you will get out of detoxification. Excess fluids in your body will speed up the process of flushing out excess toxins. Opt for purified or mineral water to ensure you're sipping the cleanest version.
- **Green Machine:** Green leafy veggies are the superheroes during detox. Spinach, kale, and chard are packed with essential nutrients and can help your body eliminate unwanted substances.
- **Berry Good Choices:** Blueberries, raspberries, and strawberries aren't just sweet treats. They're also bursting with antioxidants that can aid in the detox process.
- **Tea Time:** Herbal teas like green tea, dandelion, and nettle tea can be calming and detoxifying. They provide antioxidants and other healthful compounds beneficial during a fast.
- **Nuts About Seeds:** Flaxseeds, chia seeds, and hemp seeds are nutrient-dense and can assist in maintaining a balanced gut.
- **Friendly Fats:** Avocados and olive oil are excellent sources of healthy fats that can provide sustained energy while supporting cellular repair.

How to Get the Most Out of Your Detox During Fasting

Embarking on a fasting detox is like setting out on a transformative adventure. Over the years, I've realized that while the path to detoxification through fasting can be exhilarating, those little tweaks and personal adjustments truly make all the difference. From my journey, I've distilled some insights that can help you benefit from detox.

Firstly, always listen to your body. In my early days of fasting, I was eager to follow every advice I read. But only some things work for everyone. While some people may swear by 16-hour fasts, you might find that a 12-hour window is what your body needs. Adjust the duration based on how you feel, not just on what's trending.

Hydration is non-negotiable. While on my third detox, I noticed my energy levels soared as I increased my water intake. Water aids in flushing out toxins, so ensure you're drinking ample amounts throughout your fast. And when you break your fast, focus on nutrient-rich foods. It's tempting to dive into a hearty meal post-fast, but easing into it with a light salad or broth can be more beneficial.

Lastly, integrate mindfulness practices. Meditation and deep breathing exercises elevated the entire experience during my fasting periods. Not only do they help in centering the mind, but they also support the body's detoxification process. Your fasting detox journey is uniquely yours; embrace it with open arms, and you'll be amazed at the treasures you unearth.

MAXIMIZING DETOX DURING INTERMITTENT FASTING

Starting on your IF journey? A simple tip: stick religiously to the 12-hour gap. This time window allows your body to kick-start the detoxification process naturally. Giving your system a break enables it to recharge, reset, and commence vital repair mechanisms. But remember, consistency is key! So, set an eating window that aligns with your daily routine and honor it like a pact with a best friend.

What is the 12-hour Gap?

Diving into the specifics, the 12-hour gap in intermittent fasting refers to the period you abstain from eating. Picture it as a mini-vacation for your body. You don't consume any calories during this time, giving your digestive system a well-deserved break. This pause is more than just about avoiding food; it's a strategic pause, enabling your body to transition from using glucose for energy to tapping into stored fat. Plus, in this period, the magic of autophagy - your body's recycling system - gets activated, aiding detoxification.

"Detoxes" and "Cleanses": What You Need To Know

Detoxes and cleanses have become buzzwords, often inter-changeably used, but there's a slight difference. While both aim at eliminating toxins, detoxes are more about nourishing the body and supporting our natural detoxification pathways. Cleanses, on the other hand, often revolve around specific diets or products to expel toxins. My two cents? While considering either, ensure you're informed. Not all products or extreme diets out there are safe. Prioritize methods that focus on whole foods, hydration, and overall well-being.

Fasting & Detox Coaching

Have you ever considered having a personal guide on your fasting and detox journey? That's what fasting and detox coaching offers. Coaches provide structured plans, science-backed insights, and that emotional push when needed. On my own journey, having an expert guiding me through the maze of misinformation was enlightening. They can help you understand your body's unique requirements and tailor an approach just for you, making your fasting and detox expedition more impactful.

Best Detoxification Methods for the Body

Detoxifying doesn't have to be complex. Simple, everyday strategies can do wonders. Here's what I've gathered from my experience and research:

- **Stay Hydrated:** Water isn't just to quench your thirst; it's vital for toxin elimination.
- **Eat Whole Foods:** Lean proteins, fiber-rich foods, and healthy fats enhance your body's natural detox process.
- **Limit Processed Foods & Sugar:** Eating these foods produces unwanted toxin buildup.
- **Practice Deep Breathing:** Oxygen aids in the detoxification process.
- **Sweat It Out:** Be it through exercise or saunas, sweating helps release toxins.

YOUR ULTIMATE DETOX GUIDE

Why Detox?

- Reset your body's natural balance.
- Clear out toxins.
- Boost energy and mental clarity.
- Why do you want to detox?

Detox Basics Checklist ✅

- Stay Hydrated:

  - Drink plenty of water.
  - Avoid caffeinated and sugary drinks.

- Mind Your Diet:

  - Focus on whole foods, greens, and organic produce.
  - Minimize processed foods and sugars.

- Rest & Recovery:

  - Ensure you're getting 7-8 hours of sleep.
  - Relax and practice stress-relieving activities.

Detox Boosters - Foods & Drinks:

Lemon Water: A morning ritual for a fresh start.

Green Smoothies: Packed with vitamins and minerals.

Turmeric & Ginger Teas: Anti-inflammatory and antioxidant-rich.

Fun Fact:

Did you know fasting can help improve insulin sensitivity, boost brain function, and even reduce the risk of chronic diseases?

Safety First:

★ Listen to your body.
★ If you feel unwell, stop and consult with a healthcare professional.
★ Author's Personal Insight:

"When I started my detox journey, I was overwhelmed. But then, I realized the beauty is in the journey itself, not just the destination. Each day brought new learnings and self-awareness. Remember, it's about progress, not perfection. You've got this!"

Detox Activities:

🪷 Meditation: For a clear mind.
🧘 Walks in Nature: Breathe in fresh air and reconnect.
🛁 Warm Baths: Add Epsom salts for muscle relaxation.

DailyReflection:

How did I feel today?

What foods did I eat?

_____

How was my energy level?

_____

Navigating the Next Step

In this chapter, we've demystified the connection between detox and intermittent fasting. We've learned how fasting activates our body's natural detox mechanisms, from the wonders of autophagy to the holistic benefits it brings. Remember: enhanced immunity, mood regulation, and efficient bodily functions are all within your grasp when you combine the benefits of fasting and detox.

But the journey doesn't end here. What's the best way to fast? How can you adapt it to your unique needs? We'll tackle these questions in our next chapter, where we introduce the F.A.S.T.W.I.S.E method. This step-by-step guide is designed to make your fasting experience effective and fulfilling. Let's keep the momentum going and dive into the specifics of fasting methods!

3

F: FASTING METHODS TO CHOOSE FROM

> " *I have not only found good health, but perfect health; I have found a new state of being, a potentiality of life, a sense of lightness and cleanness and joyfulness, such as I did not know could exist in the human body.*"
>
> — UPTON SINCLAIR, THE FASTING CURE

Welcome to the first stepping stone of the F.A.S.T.W.I.S.E method: Fasting Methods. Diving into intermittent fasting, especially for women over 50, is like being presented with a smorgasbord of dining options. Do you prefer a 12-hour fast daily, or are you intrigued by the discipline of the Warrior Diet? The 5:2 method may catch your eye, or you're considering the 16:8 route. This chapter unveils the many faces of intermittent fasting, each with its unique rhythm and rewards. From Overnight Fasting to Alternate-Day Fasting, we'll explore them all, backed by inspiring success stories and tailored examples. But it doesn't stop at just picking a method. The latter part of this chapter focuses on personalizing your IF journey. Whether through apps, understanding your body's cues, or determining the optimal fasting window, you'll walk away with a plan that truly resonates with your goals and lifestyle. Let's begin this journey by looking at the many different fasting methods, ensuring you choose one that's effective and feels suitable for you.

NAVIGATING THE LANDSCAPE OF INTERMITTENT FASTING PROTOCOLS

Intermittent fasting has various styles to fit everyone's lifestyle and needs. Each method offers unique benefits, whether you're aiming to shed some weight, enhance your heart health, or guard against chronic illnesses. It's all about finding the method that's right for you. But, as with any dietary strategy, there are nuances to consider, especially for women over 50.

This section will demystify the 11 predominant IF protocols. You'll receive a thorough overview of each, ensuring a clear understanding of its structure and core principles. More critically, we will explore the pros and cons specifically for women in their post-menopausal years, a phase when the body undergoes significant changes. The insights here will help you decide which method best aligns with your health objectives and lifestyle considerations.

As we navigate these protocols, from the widely adopted 16/8 method to the more sporadic approach of spontaneous meal skipping, we must remember that every woman's journey is unique. While IF boasts numerous benefits, it's crucial to approach each method with an informed perspective, weighing the advantages against potential challenges. So, let's start on this exploration, ensuring that you're well-positioned to make a choice that celebrates and supports your well-being by the end.

1. Fast for 12 Hours a Day

One of the more straightforward and sustainable IF methods, fasting for 12 hours a day, offers a balanced window: half the day is dedicated to fasting, while the other half is for consuming meals. This approach naturally aligns with many people's lifestyles, as it can easily mirror the span from dinner to breakfast the next day, making it a subtle introduction to intermittent fasting.

✚ Pros:

- **Gentle Introduction:** This method is less intimidating and is a smooth transition into the world of fasting.
- **Flexibility:** The 12 hours can be adjusted to fit different schedules, allowing for dinner events or early breakfasts.

━ Cons:

- **Limited Fasting Benefits:** Compared to longer fasting windows, the 12-hour method might offer more limited metabolic and cellular repair advantages.
- **Potential Overeating:** Without strict guidelines on the eating window, overconsumption may occur during the 12-hour feeding period.

2. The 16:8 Method

This protocol, known commonly as the 16:8 method, requires individuals to fast for 16 hours and restrict their eating to an 8-hour window. For instance, your eating window could be between 12 pm and 8 pm. It's a popular IF method due to its ability to tap into fat reserves for energy, thus aiding in weight management.

+ Pros:

- **Enhanced Fat Burning:** A longer fasting window can lead to more pronounced metabolic benefits.
- **Convenient:** It can naturally omit breakfast, aligning with the lack of appetite of many in the morning.

− Cons:

- **Hunger Pangs:** Some may find it challenging initially, feeling hungrier in the morning.
- **Social Challenges:** Late-morning events or brunches might pose social challenges.

3. The Warrior Diet

This diet is rooted in the ancient warrior routine of long hours of fasting followed by a big feast at night. Typically, one consumes little during a 20-hour fasting window, followed by a 4-hour eating window in the evening.

+ Pros:

- **Mimics Ancient Routines:** Aligns with historical eating patterns.
- **Intense Fat Burning:** An extended fasting period can lead to significant fat loss.

− Cons:

- **Highly Restrictive:** The short eating window can be challenging to adhere to.

- **Night-time Overeating:** Risk of consuming excessive calories in the short eating period.

4. The 5:2 Method

Also known as the "Fast Diet", the 5:2 method involves eating normally for five days and reducing calorie intake (about 500-600 calories) for two non-consecutive days a week.

+ Pros:

- **Flexibility:** You can choose the two days that best fit your schedule.
- **Less Restrictive:** Only two days of calorie counting.
- **Metabolic Boost:** Potential to kickstart metabolism on low-calorie days.

— Cons:

- **Planning:** Requires planning to ensure proper nutrients on low-calorie days.
- **Energy Lows:** Reduced intake can cause fatigue or mood swings on fasting days.

5. Eat-Stop-Eat Diet

The Eat-Stop-Eat diet entails a 24-hour fast once or twice a week. You can eat your usual meals and snacks outside of these fasting periods.

+ Pros:

- **Flexibility:** Choose which days to fast based on your schedule.

- **Potential Caloric Reduction:** This can result in overall weekly calorie reduction.

— **Cons:**

- **Intensity:** 24-hour fasting can be challenging.
- **Nutrient Balance:** Risk of not getting essential nutrients if not eating balanced meals on non-fasting days.

6. The 14:10 Diet

This approach involves a 10-hour eating window and 14 hours of fasting daily. Essentially, it's a milder version of the 16:8 method.

+ Pros:

- **Gentler Introduction:** A less intense start for those new to IF.
- **Balanced Energy:** Allows for three spaced-out meals, maintaining energy levels.

— **Cons:**

- **Late Night Snacking:** This can be challenging for evening snackers.
- **Limited Fasting Benefits:** A shorter fasting duration might yield fewer benefits than longer windows.

7. Time-Restricted Fasting

Time-restricted fasting (TRF) restricts eating to certain hours of the day. It includes methods like 16:8, 14:10, etc. The focus is on the eating window rather than days of fasting.

+ Pros:

- **Consistency:** Daily routine can promote better adherence.
- **Synchronization:** Aligns eating with the body's circadian rhythm, potentially aiding sleep and metabolism.

— Cons:

- **Social Constraints:** Might interfere with social events or dinners.
- **Hunger Pangs:** Initial hunger during fasting periods until adjustment.

8. Overnight Fasting

Overnight fasting involves extending the natural fasting period that occurs during sleep. Typically, this means finishing dinner early in the evening and not eating again until breakfast, ensuring a fasting window of around 12 hours or more.

+ Pros:

- **Natural Rhythm:** Aligns with the body's circadian rhythm, potentially promoting better sleep and metabolism.
- **Ease of Adoption:** Less disruptive since a significant portion of the fast occurs during sleep.

— **Cons:**

- **Limited Evening Flexibility:** Can conflict with late dinners or social events.
- **Milder Benefits:** Compared to longer fasts, benefits might be more subtle.

9. 23/1 Fast

The 23/1 fast, often called the "OMAD" (One Meal A Day) diet, requires adherents to fast for 23 hours, leaving just a 1-hour eating window. During this hour, individuals consume their daily caloric intake in a single meal.

+ Pros:

- **Simplified Meal Planning:** Only planning and preparing one meal can be convenient.
- **Potent Metabolic Benefits:** An extended fasting period can enhance fat-burning and improve insulin sensitivity.

— **Cons:**

- **Intense Hunger:** A prolonged fasting window can be challenging, leading to intense hunger pangs.
- **Overeating Risk:** The pressure to consume a day's worth of calories in an hour might lead to overindulgence.

10. Whole-Day Fasting

A complete 24-hour cycle without food defines whole-day fasting, usually from one night's dinner to the subsequent evening.

This approach should involve consuming water, tea, or other non-caloric beverages during the fasting window.

+ Pros:

- **Enhanced Cellular Repair:** A longer fast can trigger autophagy, aiding cellular clean-up.
- **Flexibility:** Allows occasional indulgences on non-fasting days.

− Cons:

- **Challenging:** A whole day without food can be mentally and physically demanding.
- **Potential Nutrient Deficiency:** Regularly missing out on a day's worth of nutrients might require careful dietary planning.

11. Alternate-Day Fasting

Alternate-day fasting involves cycling between regular eating and fasting. You spend one day eating normally, and the next is either fully fasting or consuming very few calories.

+ Pros:

- **Weight Management:** This method has shown effective weight loss results for many.
- **Metabolic Health:** It can improve markers like blood sugar and cholesterol levels.

− Cons:

- **Consistency Issues:** Alternating days can make maintaining a consistent eating routine harder.

- **Social Implications:** Fasting every other day can interfere with social meals and events.

TAILORING INTERMITTENT FASTING TO YOUR LIFESTYLE

As women step gracefully into their 50s, the need for a health routine that resonates with their unique body requirements becomes paramount. This section, intersecting at the crossroads of modern technology and age-old fasting wisdom, focuses on personalizing Intermittent Fasting to the distinctive needs of women over 50. The symphony of metabolism, lifestyle, and well-being doesn't play the same tune for everyone. Therefore, it's essential to understand that while the principles of IF remain universal, the application can be as varied as the individuals embracing it. Explore different fasting schedules to find a routine that best suits your unique lifestyle. By integrating advanced tools like Lumen and utilizing top-rated fasting apps, you'll be well on your way to a tailored fasting journey. Intermittent fasting is about matching your eating schedule with your body's natural rhythms. Set up a fasting plan that works with your metabolism, identify the most fitting fasting windows, and consider factors that ensure your chosen schedule complements your lifestyle. By doing so, you can make fasting work for you and reap all the fantastic rewards it has to offer.

Best Intermittent Fasting Apps for Weight Loss

In today's digital age, technology amplifies the potency of Intermittent Fasting by giving you tools that fit right into your pocket. Navigating your IF journey becomes more streamlined, focused, and achievable with the right apps. Here are some top contenders:

- **Zero:** A crowd-favorite, Zero offers user-friendly interfaces, tracking for various fasting methods, and a journal feature to note your experiences, ensuring your journey is not just effective but also reflective.
- **FastHabit:** Highlighting its flexibility, FastHabit allows you to set your fasting and eating windows, sends reminders, and offers a glance at your progress over weeks.
- **Life Fasting Tracker:** A comprehensive tool, this app tracks your fasting windows and allows social connections. Share your progress with friends or join groups for added motivation.
- **BodyFast:** More than just a tracker, BodyFast suggests personalized fasting plans based on your input data, merging tech with a personal touch.
- **Simple:** As the name implies, it's all about simplicity. Simple is a holistic approach to IF with hydration reminders, meal logging, and even advice on what foods to consume.

Choosing an app is more than just downloading software; it's about finding a digital companion that aligns with your IF goals. Each app offers unique features, but all aim to support and enhance your weight loss journey with intermittent fasting.

CRAFTING A PERSONALIZED INTERMITTENT FASTING SCHEDULE

The beauty of IF is its flexibility. Here's how to tailor it to reflect the unique essence of every vibrant woman over 50:

1. Assessing Your Lifestyle and Health Needs: Understanding your health goals and daily routine before diving into a fasting routine. Are you seeking improved brain function, enhanced metabolism, or weight loss? Aligning your goals with your fasting schedule is paramount.

2. Discovering Your Fasting Window: A successful fasting journey hinges on finding the optimal window that complements your body's natural rhythm. Start with shorter fasting intervals, like 12 hours, and gradually increase the duration, observing how your body responds.

3. Utilizing Cutting-Edge Tools: Embrace technology like Lumen, a revolutionary device that gauges your metabolism using breath analysis. By determining whether your body is burning fats or carbs, Lumen offers invaluable insights, helping you adjust your fasting periods for maximum benefit.

4. Seek Feedback and Adjust: Listen to your body. If you feel vibrant and energized, you're on the right track. If fatigue sets in, consider tweaking your schedule. The key is fluidity and adjustment.

Crafting the perfect IF schedule is both a science and a personal journey. By grounding your approach in sound physiological understanding and data-driven strategies, you can harness the most effective elements of fasting. But remember, it's not just about metrics. It's about how you feel and respond to the regimen as a vibrant woman over 50. Merging scientific insights with your unique body responses and personal goals ensures a path to success that feels right and enhances your overall well-being.

Choosing Your Perfect Fasting Rhythm: Essential Factors to Consider

Picking the proper intermittent fasting schedule is pivotal for sustained success. Here are some handy tips to keep in mind when selecting your perfect fasting match:

Personal Lifestyle & Routine: Your daily activities are pivotal in determining your fasting schedule. A night-time fasting routine may be ideal if you're an early riser who likes a hearty breakfast before the day begins. On the other hand, if evenings are reserved for social activities or dinners, consider morning fasts. It's about integrating fasting seamlessly into your routine, ensuring it complements rather than disrupts your day.

Health Goals: The purpose behind your fasting can significantly influence the regimen you adopt. Consistent daily fasts offer the desired calorie restriction if you aim for weight loss. If boosting metabolic health is the target, extended fasts can push the body to optimize energy utilization. For those seeking cognitive improvements, research suggests regular shorter fasts can potentially encourage brain-derived neurotrophic factors.

Physical Responses: As unique as our fingerprints, our body's reaction to fasting varies. It's vital to observe and listen to your body. Some might find they're more energetic and focused during a 16:8 fasting routine. In contrast, others might discover that alternate-day fasting brings out their best. It's a journey of understanding your body's cues and feedback.

Medical History: Your past and current health conditions play a decisive role. For instance, someone with a history of eating disorders should approach IF with caution. Similarly, medications, especially those that need food intake, can impact when and how you should fast. Always prioritize your health and consult a healthcare professional when introducing new dietary practices.

Consistency is Key: While it's tempting to jump between various fasting schedules, it's the consistency that usually delivers the magic. Stick to it once you've found a rhythm that resonates with you and brings the desired results. Establishing a regular pattern trains your body and mind, enhancing the bene-fits and smoothing the journey.

SUCCESSES WITH INTERMITTENT FASTING

Across the globe, women in their prime years have been experi-encing the transformative power of Intermittent Fasting. Their success stories, scattered across the web, are a testament to the versatility and efficacy of this approach.

One woman struggling with post-menopausal weight gain adopted the 16:8 fasting routine. In doing so, she not only managed to shed those persistent pounds but also found a renewed sense of vitality and flexibility. "I was skeptical when I started fasting, but the results made it clear - it was the best decision of my life! I've never felt better!" Cory S., New York.

Another professional facing the stresses of a demanding career turned to the 5:2 method. The outcome was a clear head, better focus, and a notable reduction in menopausal symptoms. "When my work started to suffer, I knew it was time for a change. IF has kept me focused and on track, and my clients love me for it!" Jeannette R., Ohio.

Elsewhere, a grandmother wishing to keep up with her ener-getic grandkids chose alternate-day fasting. Her reward was not just in weight management, but in the increased energy and improved health she enjoyed. "I have more energy now to play with my grandkids, and that's the most important thing for me!" Esther L., Toronto.

And in another corner of the globe, a dedicated fitness coach, feeling the strains of age on her routine, turned to time-restricted fasting. The results were not just weight loss but an enhancement in her strength and training performance. "Exercise and IF go hand-in-hand for me. Both require a unique mindfulness that keeps me focused and helps me stay strong and balanced." Romena R., Manilla.

Such inspiring accounts drove my curiosity, leading me on a personal journey of exploration with IF. After experimenting with various methods, I found a rhythm that suited my body and lifestyle, offering me renewed energy, improved sleep, and a handle on post-menopausal challenges. These stories, along with my own, remind me that with the right approach, IF can be tailored to fit any individual's needs. Hearing these uplifting stories pushed me to try IF myself. I tried different methods and eventually found one that worked well for me, offering me renewed energy, improved sleep, and helped with post-menopausal issues. These stories, along with my own, remind me that with the right approach, IF can be tailored to fit any individual's needs.

Finding My Rhythm with IF

Navigating the world of Intermittent Fasting felt much like setting sail into uncharted waters. With the abundance of information available and many methods to choose from, the initial step was both exhilarating and a tad overwhelming. But the remarkable transformations of other women, combined with my innate drive, propelled me forward.

To chart my course, I began by exploring several fasting apps. Zero and FastHabit offered comprehensive tracking tools, while Life Fasting Tracker provided a supportive community of like-minded fasters. Simple's interface was user-friendly, emphasizing the nuances of IF. However, during this exploration, I stumbled upon Lumen, a metabolic measurement tool. The handheld device seemed almost futuristic – gauging metabolism through breath analysis. I could receive real-time feedback using Lumen, allowing me to adjust my fasting and nutrition strategy daily. It became an invaluable tool on my journey, shedding light on how my body responded to various IF protocols.

Armed with technology and determination, I began trying different methods. The 16:8 approach initially seemed promising, but I struggled with evening hunger pangs. The 5:2 method offered more flexibility, but the calorie-restricted days proved challenging for my active lifestyle. Time-restricted fasting ultimately resonated with me, offering a balanced blend of discipline and freedom.

Throughout my journey, constant self-awareness was pivotal. By monitoring physical responses and aligning them with the insights from Lumen, I sculpted an IF regimen tailored harmoniously to my needs. The benefits became palpable as days turned to weeks – heightened energy, stabilized mood swings, improved sleep quality, and a renewed sense of vitality.

Reflecting upon my experience, it becomes evident that while IF's principles remain consistent, its application is profoundly personal. Everyone's path might vary, but with determination, the right advice, and some helpful tools, anyone can create their way to better health and renewal.

Embracing Your Unique IF Journey

This chapter explored the world of Intermittent Fasting, a practice proving to be transformative for countless women over 50. We've scoured the various fasting methods available, understanding that there isn't a one-size-fits-all approach. The true power of IF lies in its flexibility and adaptability to fit each individual's unique needs, lifestyle, and health goals. Remember, every journey starts with understanding, and armed with knowledge, you can personalize your IF routine, optimize your metabolic health, and carve a path toward rejuvenation and vitality.

However, merely knowing the methods is only half the battle. As we step into the next chapter, we'll embark on a journey to truly 'adapt'—which fittingly is the "A" in our F.A.S.T.W.I.S.E. framework. Preparing for the IF lifestyle is more than just choosing a fasting schedule; it's about setting the stage for seamless integration into your daily life. Join me as we look into the nuances of adaptation, ensuring that your IF journey is not just effective but also sustainable and harmonious with your vibrant life over 50.

4

A: ADAPTATION AND PREPARING FOR THE IF LIFESTYLE

> *"Intermittent fasting is a lifestyle. It isn't something that you start today and then end when you get to some arbitrary "goal weight." Something you start and then stop is a DIET. Intermittent fasting isn't a diet – as I said, it's a lifestyle."*

— GIN STEPHENS

Unlike the countless diets that come and go, leaving us in cycles of joy and disappointment, intermittent fasting is a commitment to yourself. It's not just a temporary fix but a long-term strategy encouraging women over 50 to embrace a more vibrant, healthier version of themselves. Before starting on this path, it's imperative to be fully armed, both mentally and physically. You wouldn't set sail on an uncharted journey without a compass, would you? Similarly, it is necessary to be thoroughly prepared for the IF journey.

In this chapter, we'll unravel the layers of mental and physical groundwork essential for your upcoming IF voyage. Next, we will look at the psychological and physical preparation necessary for your forthcoming journey in IF. We'll pick a day to start your fast, understand the medical considerations unique to women in their golden years, and embark on the rewarding task of setting clear, achievable goals. By exploring these topics, you give yourself the best chance for success and can start your intermittent fast with the proper knowledge and preparation.

LAYING THE GROUNDWORK: MIND AND BODY ALIGNMENT FOR FASTING

Your intermittent fasting journey demands more than just setting a timer and waiting for it to go off. It's about harmonizing both your mind and body for the profound change that lies ahead. This alignment of mental and physical facets ensures your fasting experience is successful and fulfilling.

Mental and Physical Preparation

Your body is an intricate system, and introducing it to the intermittent fasting regimen should be gradual. Think of it as tuning a musical instrument: start gently and adjust until you hit the perfect note. Start with shorter fasting intervals, like 10 hours, and progressively extend them to longer periods, such as 16 hours. This incremental approach not only eases your body into the fasting rhythm but also allows your mind to adapt without feeling overwhelmed.

Hydration is paramount. Make water and calorie-free beverages like herbal teas your constant companions. This not only keeps thirst at bay but also helps suppress hunger pangs during fasting periods. Equally important is the nourishment you provide during your eating window. Prioritize nutrient-dense foods to ensure you're fueling your body with the necessary vitamins and minerals.

Training the mind is as critical as preparing the body. Redirecting thoughts when hunger creeps in can be a powerful tool. Instead of thinking about food during fasting, channel your focus towards other activities. This mental diversion will build resilience over time. Remember, consistency is the key to fostering a positive mindset.

Intensive exercise during fasting periods might sound tempting, but it's best to tread lightly. Listen to your body; if you choose to exercise, keep it moderate. Lastly, don't let the number of fasting methods overwhelm you. Select a strategy that aligns best with your lifestyle and comfort, whether alternate-day fasting, the 5:2 approach, or daily time-restricted fasting. And remember, you can always switch to a new method anytime! If something doesn't feel right, take a step back and start again.

Choose-Your-Day Fasting: Tailoring Fasting to Your Lifestyle

Integrating intermittent fasting into your life doesn't mean fitting your life around the fasting schedule but rather fitting fasting into your existing life. That's the beauty of Choose-Your-Day Fasting. Here, we mold the fasting routine to match the rhythm of your day-to-day activities, ensuring it complements rather than conflicts with your commitments.

When I began my intermittent fasting journey, I quickly realized there were more practical approaches than a fixed schedule. There were days filled with family gatherings, social events, and work meetings that made fasting challenging. I decided to tailor my fasting around these events. If I knew a special event was approaching, I would adjust my fasting schedule to accommodate it. It was crucial to remember that while fasting is a commitment, it doesn't require turning down invitations or missing out on memorable moments.

What Are the Rules of Intermittent Fasting?

Intermittent fasting, at its core, is a dietary pattern that shifts between fasting and eating. This practice doesn't so much focus on the types of food you eat but rather on when you eat. To help you navigate the waters of intermittent fasting, here's a breakdown:

- **Choose a Fasting Window:** Determine a fasting duration that aligns with your goals and lifestyle. This window can range from 12 to 20 hours. During this time, keep caloric intake to a minimum.
- **Stick to Non-Caloric Drinks:** Avoid any food or beverages with calories during the fasting period. Stick to water, black coffee, or tea to maintain hydration without interrupting the fast.
- **Nutritionally Balanced Meals:** When your eating window arrives, focus on nourishing, balanced meals. While it might be tempting, avoid the urge to overeat. It's about feeding the body efficiently, not excessively.
- **Consistency is Key:** Regularity in your eating pattern helps in adapting to intermittent fasting. Maintain a predictable routine to make the transition smoother.
- **Exercise and Supplements:** Moderate exercise complements fasting, but tuning into your body's signals is essential. If needed, consider supplements to compensate for any nutritional shortfalls.
- **Stay Relaxed:** This journey is about enhancing your life, not adding stress. Enjoy the process, and remember the approach is flexible.

Adjusting to Intermittent Fasting

As you venture into intermittent fasting, remember that there are multiple methods to explore, like the 16/8 method, Eat-Stop-Eat, or the 5:2 diet. Selecting the right one depends on your comfort, needs, and objectives.

The initial days might seem overwhelming. The body and mind will need time to adjust to this new rhythm. Begin by identifying which part of the day you naturally feel less inclined to eat. For some, skipping breakfast is more manageable, while others prefer skipping dinner.

My advice? Stay patient and give yourself grace. The adaptation phase varies for everyone. With time and persistence, intermittent fasting will soon feel like a natural extension of your lifestyle, enhancing your health journey.

MEDICAL CONSIDERATIONS: THE HEALTH IMPACTS OF INTERMITTENT FASTING

Understanding the potential medical implications of intermittent fasting is crucial. While many opt for intermittent fasting for weight management or lifestyle reasons, emerging research suggests it also offers significant health benefits.

Heart disease, often dubbed the "silent killer," remains a leading cause of death globally. Remarkably, intermittent fasting has been shown to minimize various heart disease risk factors, including obesity, cholesterol, blood pressure, and insulin resistance. But its potential benefits continue beyond there. The practice has also been linked to reduced inflammation, improved blood sugar control, and even support for neurodegenerative conditions like Parkinson's disease. Furthermore, studies hint at its role in enhancing cognitive functions, such as working memory in animals and verbal memory in humans.

Navigating the world of nutrition and health can be complex. Yet, with the right knowledge, intermittent fasting can be a tool that reshapes your body and bolsters your overall health. This section will explore how intermittent fasting interacts with various medical conditions. We will also guide readers through the ideal food and drink selections during fasting periods, ensuring an understanding of its safety implications. With this information, you will be well-armed to decide whether intermittent fasting is the right choice for your health goals.

7 Medical Conditions That Intermittent Fasting May Help

The allure of intermittent fasting goes beyond its potential for weight management. Recent studies have unveiled its promising impact on a spectrum of health conditions. While the idea of consciously limiting food intake for specified hours might seem like a modern trend, it's deeply rooted in ancient practices, and now science is catching up. Next, we'll discuss how intermittent fasting can help with seven common medical issues. By understanding its role in each of these ailments, you can make an informed choice about integrating IF into their wellness journey.

1. Insulin Resistance:

Insulin resistance occurs when cells don't respond efficiently to insulin, a hormone that regulates blood sugar. Intermittent fasting can enhance the body's sensitivity to insulin. By imposing regular short-term fasts, IF reduces blood sugar levels, ensuring that cells can use insulin more effectively, thus reducing the risk of progressing to more severe conditions like Type 2 Diabetes.

2. Type 2 Diabetes:

Characterized by high blood sugar and insulin resistance, Type 2 Diabetes can significantly benefit from intermittent fasting. IF helps regulate blood sugar levels, decreasing the need for insulin. In many instances, this regulation can aid in managing and reversing some aspects of the condition.

3. PCOS:

Polycystic Ovary Syndrome (PCOS) is a hormonal disorder in women. Intermittent fasting, by regulating insulin levels and reducing insulin resistance - a common factor in PCOS - may alleviate some symptoms and improve hormonal balance.

4. Obesity:

At its core, intermittent fasting can create a caloric deficit essential for weight loss. Beyond this, IF influences metabolic pathways and hormones, optimizing fat burn and lean muscle preservation, making it an effective tool against obesity.

5. Cardiovascular Disease:

Heart health remains a global concern. Intermittent fasting has shown potential in lowering risk factors like high blood pressure, cholesterol levels, triglycerides, and inflammatory markers, all of which are pivotal in warding off cardiovascular diseases.

6. Gastrointestinal Health:

Regular breaks from eating, as facilitated by intermittent fasting, can give the digestive system a much-needed rest. These breaks can improve gut motility and health, reducing symptoms like bloating, constipation, and irregular bowel movements.

7. Neurodegenerative Disorders:

There's growing evidence that intermittent fasting can support brain health. By reducing oxidative stress and inflammation, IF might play a role in staving off neurodegenerative conditions such as Alzheimer's and Parkinson's diseases.

The Science Behind Intermittent Fasting: From Metabolism to Medical Testing

Intermittent fasting is more than just a dietary regimen; it's an integration of biology, circadian rhythm, and metabolic pathways, all of which play a role in overall health. Let's explore the science-backed reasons for its increasing popularity.

1. Intermittent Fasting Optimizes Circadian Metabolism:

Our body operates on a natural circadian rhythm, an internal clock regulating sleep-wake cycles and metabolic processes. IF aligns with this rhythm, supporting a harmonious synchronization between food intake and metabolic functions. This results in optimized energy utilization and promotes cellular repair, primarily during fasting.

2. Reducing Oxidative Stress:

Oxidative stress, caused by an imbalance between free radicals and antioxidants, can damage cells and DNA. The body becomes more resilient to oxidative stress with IF, possibly diminishing chronic disease risks.

3. Improved Insulin Sensitivity:

By periodically restricting calorie intake, IF improves insulin responsiveness, ensuring cells absorb glucose effectively from the bloodstream. This reduction in insulin resistance is pivotal in managing and even preventing conditions like Type 2 diabetes.

Labs to Consider for Patients on Intermittent Fasting:

Monitoring physiological responses is crucial for practicing IF, especially to tailor the approach to individual health needs. If you are starting IF, talk to your doctor about monitoring these key health indicators through regular blood work checks:

- **Fasting Glucose:** Measures blood sugar levels after fasting, highlighting the body's glucose regulation capabilities.
- **Insulin Levels:** Monitors the amount of insulin, providing insights into pancreatic function and insulin resistance.
- **HbA1c:** Gives a long-term picture of blood sugar levels, representing an average over 2-3 months. It's particularly beneficial for those at risk for diabetes.
- **Continuous Glucose Monitor:** Provides real-time, constant glucose monitoring. This data gives healthcare

professionals an understanding of how diet and lifestyle cause fluctuations in sugar levels throughout the day.

- **Comprehensive Female Hormones Panel:** Especially pertinent for women over 50, this test examines hormone levels, which dietary patterns, including IF, can influence.
- **Boston Heart Lifestyle Panel:** This test covers numerous cardiovascular risk factors to give patients a thorough overview of their heart and cardiovascular system health.
- **Comprehensive Stool Test:** The stool test examines a stool sample for those who want a better understanding of their gut health. This test gives insight into your digestive function and gut microbiome balance, showing any potential signs of inflammation.

Intermittent Fasting: Not a One Size Fits All Solution

Intermittent fasting offers numerous health benefits, but it is only suitable for some. While many have found success with this dietary approach, there are specific situations where IF might not be the best choice. Here's a rundown of conditions or scenarios where pausing or rethinking the decision to take on intermittent fasting is recommended.

- **Sleep Concerns:** If you're grappling with sleep problems, IF might exacerbate them. Sleep and nutrition are closely linked, and fasting can sometimes disrupt sleep patterns for some individuals.
- **History of Disordered Eating:** Individuals with a past of disordered eating or diagnosed eating disorders should approach IF with caution. The restrictive nature might trigger old habits or detrimental behaviors.

- **Intensive Physical Training:** Those involved in rigorous training or looking to gain muscle might find the restricted eating window limiting, potentially hampering their nutritional and energy needs.
- **Digestive Troubles:** If you've got digestion issues, the prolonged fasting periods may exacerbate symptoms or discomfort.
- **Jobs Demanding Sharp Focus:** Professions requiring intense concentration might be compromised if your energy levels or focus dips during fasting windows.
- **Diabetes:** People with diabetes, particularly those on insulin or specific medications, must be cautious, as IF can affect blood sugar levels.
- **Pregnancy or Breastfeeding:** Sufficient nutrition is necessary during this time. It's crucial to ensure consistent and adequate caloric intake for both mother and child.
- **Medications and Food:** If you're on medication that mandates consumption with food, IF might be challenging or unsafe.
- **Weak Immune System or Cancer:** IF could further weaken the immune system, making it unsuitable for those already compromised or undergoing cancer treatments.
- **Inflexible Lifestyle:** For some, work schedules, social commitments, or family routines can't accommodate strict eating windows. Choosing a dietary approach that integrates seamlessly with your lifestyle is essential.
- **Personal Preference:** Ultimately, the decision lies with individual preference. If you're uncomfortable or wish to eat outside a designated time frame, IF might not be your cup of tea.

As always, it's paramount to consult with a healthcare professional before starting or stopping any dietary regimen, especially if you fall into one of the categories above. Remember, the best dietary plan is the one tailored to an individual's unique needs and circumstances.

GOAL-SETTING FOR YOUR INTERMITTENT FASTING JOURNEY

For every transformative journey, the first step isn't just to take action but to set a clear and compelling destination. While it is a potent tool for enhancing health, intermittent fasting is not just a method but a journey, especially for women over 50. With the unique challenges and strengths that come with age, diving into this world without a roadmap can feel overwhelming.

The art of goal setting goes beyond the simple desire to lose weight or boost metabolism. It's about setting intentions that resonate deeply with one's life vision, aligning with the transformative 29-day journey. The power of a well-defined goal lies not just in the achievement but in the process, the enlightenment, and the personal growth.

For women over 50, understanding the 'why' behind this intermittent fasting journey becomes a catalyst for motivation. It's not about fitting into a specific mold but embracing a health-conscious lifestyle that celebrates the wisdom of our years. As we explore this next step, we will motivate you to set your goals. Strong goals will keep you on track and push you further toward success.

How to Set and Get Your Intermittent Fasting Goals

You are starting on a journey that is one bold step towards a healthier you. With the right intentions set, your journey becomes more than an attempt; it transforms into a mission. Having reasonable goals is like having a map to success. Goals aren't just checkpoints; they help keep you motivated, especially on tough days. Goals aren't just markers but powerful motivators that keep your momentum alive, even on challenging days.

Enter the SMART goal-setting method – a proven technique that brings clarity and actionable steps to any ambition.

- **Specific:** Your fasting goal should be clear and precise. Instead of saying, "I want to lose weight," specify it like, "I aim to lose 10 pounds within two months through intermittent fasting."
- **Measurable:** Ensure that your goal can be tracked and evaluated. For instance, if your goal is to fast for 16 hours a day, you can easily measure this by noting your start and end times.
- **Achievable:** While ambition is crucial, setting goals that are too challenging can lead to discouragement. Choose goals that stretch you but remain within the realm of possibility. Consider starting with a 12-hour fasting window before leaping to a more extended period.
- **Relevant:** Your fasting goals should align with your health and lifestyle objectives. If you're aiming for improved mental clarity or reduced inflammation, ensure your intermittent fasting style supports these outcomes.
- **Time-bound:** When do you want to achieve your goal? You may be gearing up for a milestone birthday or another significant event. Setting a timeline adds urgency and commitment to your plan.

Tips for Starting Your Intermittent Fasting Journey

Whether seeking better health, weight loss, or an energy boost, this journey is about aligning your eating patterns with your unique goals. The following tips break down the essentials to kickstart your fasting journey, ensuring you approach it with clarity, confidence, and a plan that works best for you.

- **Identify Personal Goals:** Before you dive into intermittent fasting, ask yourself: Why am I doing this? You may be aiming for weight loss, improved metabolic health, or just exploring a new way to feel energized. Knowing your "why" will anchor your journey and keep you focused.
- **Pick the Method:** Intermittent fasting isn't one-size-fits-all. Some people opt for the 16/8 method (16 hours of fasting and an 8-hour eating window). In contrast, others might use the 5:2 method (eat normally for five days and significantly reduce calories for two non-consecutive days). Choose what fits best with your lifestyle and feels sustainable for you.
- **Figure Out Calorie Needs:** To maintain, lose, or even gain weight while on intermittent fasting, you must know how many calories your body requires daily. Online calculators or consultations with nutritionists can provide an estimate based on your age, gender, activity level, and goals.
- **Draft a Meal Plan:** Plan your meals once you know your calorie needs. While intermittent fasting isn't strictly about what you eat, planning can ensure a balanced intake of proteins, fats, and carbohydrates, making your eating window more effective and ensuring you're nourishing your body. Our 29-Day Meal Plan is the perfect guide for your IF routine. It

takes the guesswork out of what to eat and provides you with a clear plan of what to eat to nourish your body best. This handy guide should become your constant reference, ensuring you always feel full and satisfied.

Make the Calories Count:

It's not just about the number of calories; it's about their quality. Ensure that you fill your plate with an abundance of nutrient-dense foods. These will provide you with all the essential vitamins and minerals you require. Stock up on vegetables, lean proteins, and healthy fats, and remove processed options from your diet. When you make every calorie count, you can optimize the benefits that fasting can provide.

My Personal Dive into Intermittent Fasting

Have you ever wondered how changing when you eat, not just what you eat, can transform your health and leave you feeling younger and more vibrant? When I first spotted an article about intermittent fasting in a women's health magazine, I couldn't contain my curiosity. Reading about many women experiencing its benefits made me wonder if it might fit me well.

It wasn't just the prospect of shedding some pounds that drew me in. I was intrigued by the numerous health advantages it offers. Who wouldn't want sharper mental focus, less inflammation, and a burst of vitality?

Picking the right fasting style for me was a challenging decision. I took my time, did my homework, and considered which option best suited my lifestyle. Eventually, I settled on a daily time-restricted plan, confining my meals to a 10-hour window each day.

Those first days definitely weren't a walk in the park. The grumbles of my stomach were hard to ignore. But as the days turned into weeks, I felt a noticeable shift. I woke up with a clearer head, my afternoon fatigue was less, and my occasional joint pains seemed to ease.

Yet the journey was about more than just physical changes. It nudged me to be more thoughtful about my diet. I started paying more attention to the quality of my meals, not just the timing. I thought about how every bite I ate would benefit my body.

It wasn't all smooth sailing; sometimes, I would get thrown off track. Social events were challenging, and I had my fair share of raised eyebrows from friends and loved ones. But through it all, I stayed grounded in my initial reasons for trying intermittent fasting.

Looking back, this wasn't just about an eating schedule. It was a lesson in self-control, awareness, and truly tuning into my body's needs. Despite all its ups and downs, it's a journey I'm grateful for.

If you are thinking about starting IF, I support you wholeheartedly. There will be bumps along the way, but overcoming these challenges makes the journey worthwhile. If I can do it, you can too! And once you start, I can guarantee you will be as hooked as I am!

PREPARING FOR YOUR INTERMITTENT FASTING JOURNEY

○ *Grocery Shopping List:*

Non-Starchy Vegetables:

- Broccoli
- Spinach
- Kale
- Bell peppers
- Zucchini
- Cauliflower

High Fiber Foods:

- Chia seeds
- Flaxseeds
- Whole grains like quinoa and oats
- Lentils
- Beans
- Berries (raspberries, blackberries)

Quality Proteins:

- Lean meats (chicken, turkey)
- Fish (especially fatty fish like salmon)
- Eggs
- Tofu and tempeh for vegetarians

Healthy Fats:

- Avocados
- Olive oil
- Nuts (almonds, walnuts)
- Seeds (pumpkin seeds, sunflower seeds)
- Coconut oil

○ *Purge Your Pantry:*

Remove:

- Candy and sugary snacks
- Chips and processed salty snacks
- Processed foods with preservatives and artificial ingredients
- Sugary drinks and sodas
- High caffeine beverages

Limit:

- Alcohol (especially sugary cocktails or high-calorie beers)
- Excess caffeinated drinks like coffee (stick to 1-2 cups daily)

○ *Exercise Tips:*

- **Keep it Moderate:** Intense workouts might be challenging initially during your fasting window. Opt for light to moderate activities like walking, jogging, or low-impact aerobics.

- **Stay Hydrated:** Keep your water bottle handy whether you're working out. Proper hydration can help stave off hunger pangs.
- **Listen to Your Body:** Don't push too hard if you feel light-headed or overly tired. Adjust your exercise routine accordingly.

○ *Mental Preparation:*

- **Understanding Why:** Reflect on why you're starting intermittent fasting. Jot down the health benefits you hope to achieve.
- **Stay Informed:** Familiarize yourself with potential challenges. Knowledge can help address any apprehensions.
- **Mindful Eating:** Focus on the quality of food you consume, not just the quantity. Treasure each meal as a nourishment opportunity.
- **Positivity Journal:** Keep a journal to note positive feelings, changes, and experiences during the fasting journey. It can act as motivation during challenging times.
- **Support System:** Share your intentions with close friends or family. Their support can be invaluable; they might even join you in your journey!

YOUR JOURNEY'S FOUNDATION

As we wrap up this chapter, reflecting on the cornerstones that will guide your intermittent fasting journey is crucial. We've delved deep into understanding the "why" behind intermittent fasting, setting solid, achievable goals, preparing our body and mind for the fasting regimen, and learning from personal experiences. These are your anchors, ensuring you remain centered and on track.

Next up, we'll tackle a crucial topic: Nutrition. In the next chapter, "Setting up the Body for Success with Nutrition," we'll focus on the 'S' from our F.A.S.T.W.I.S.E framework. Nutrition is more than just choosing the right foods. It's also about the timing and approach, especially when fasting. We'll show you how to make good food choices and use meal planning to maximize your fasting plan. By matching fasting with proper nutrition, every meal becomes a step closer to achieving your goals.

MAKE A DIFFERENCE WITH YOUR REVIEW

UNLOCK THE POWER OF GENEROSITY

"Kindness is a language which the deaf can hear and the blind can see."

— MARK TWAIN

Hey there! Did you know people who give without expecting anything in return tend to be happier and healthier? That's a pretty neat fact, isn't it? Well, I've got a little favor to ask of you...

Would you be willing to help someone you've never met, without expecting a thank you?

Who is this mystery person, you wonder? They're a lot like you. Remember when you first started thinking about your health and wellness, feeling a bit lost and needing guidance? That's them.

Our big goal with "The Ultimate Guide to Intermittent Fasting for Women Over 50" is to make health and happiness easy for everyone. Everything I do is about reaching that goal. But to really make it happen, we need to reach...well, everyone!

That's where your superpower comes in. Believe it or not, most people decide on a book by its cover (and its reviews). So, here's my request on behalf of a wonderful person out there you've never met:

Could you please leave a review for this book?

It won't cost you a dime and takes less than a minute, but your words could change someone's life. Your review might help...

- ...another wonderful lady find the energy to play with her grandkids.
- ...a friend to dance like nobody's watching in her living room.
- ...someone to tackle their dreams with newfound zest.

Feeling good and making a difference is just a review away. Here's how you can do it:

Simply scan the QR code below to leave your review:

If you love the idea of helping someone out there, even if you'll never meet them, then you're awesome! Welcome to the club. You're one of us.

I'm super excited to help you find more energy, better health, and lots of happiness. Wait until you see the tips and tricks I've got for you in the next chapters.

Thank you from the bottom of my heart. Now, let's get back to our journey of feeling great.

Your biggest fan, Francis Harding

PS - Here's a fun thought: If you share something valuable with someone, it makes you more valuable in their eyes. If you think this book could help someone you know, why not share it with them?

5

S: SETTING UP YOUR BODY FOR SUCCESS WITH NUTRITIOUS MEALS

> *"You are what you eat - so don't be fast, cheap, easy or fake."*

— UNKNOWN AUTHOR

When I started my journey with intermittent fasting, I was like many of you. I had high hopes, I felt a bit skeptical, but more than anything else, I was eager for results. However, one of the things that I quickly realized was that while timing mattered, the food I ate during my eating window mattered even more. The Intermittent fasting journey isn't just about when we eat; it's also very much about the foods we fuel our bodies with.

The purpose of this next part of the book is simple, and yet it may be the most important chapter you will read. Together, we will explore how choosing the right foods to nourish your body can mean the difference between success and failure in our intermittent fasting experience. In my journey, I found that the better I ate, the better I felt. My focus quickly shifted from just wanting to lose weight to enjoying the feeling of being more energetic, awake, and alert. Nutritious meals became my best friend. They gave me the energy I needed to feel energized all day, even during my fasting hours. I want all of you to have the same successful experience that I have had. In the following pages, I will give you all the knowledge you will need to make the best food choices so that, just like me, you can feel your best while on this intermittent fasting journey. Bon appetit!

THE IMPORTANCE OF GOOD NUTRITION WHEN FASTING

The foods you eat play a critical role in your overall health. They give your body vitamins, minerals, and the fuel required to power you through your busy days. While IF is an excellent tool to help you manage your eating times, ensuring that the food you consume during these eating windows is nutrient-rich makes all the difference. This nourishment will determine how you feel and the level of success you experience in reaching your IF goals.

Foods to Help Nourish Your Body

These nutrient-rich foods can play a vital role in enhancing how effective your intermittent fasting regimen is. These foods are especially beneficial for women over 50. Our nutritional needs change as we age, and we can reap the benefits of including more nutrient-dense, whole foods in our diet.

- **Eggs:** Often called nature's multivitamin, eggs are a nutritional powerhouse. They come packed with high-quality proteins, essential for muscle maintenance and growth. Beyond protein, they contain crucial vitamins such as B12, D, A, and E. The fat content in eggs is rich in Omega-3s, particularly in the more wholesome, pasture-raised varieties. Eggs also contain choline, which helps with liver function and brain development, while selenium is a powerful antioxidant that works hard to protect our cells.

- **Fish and Seafood:** Beyond being a rich source of high-quality protein, fish and seafood offer some of the best sources of Omega-3 fatty acids – known for their anti-inflammatory properties. Regularly eating seafood can ward off chronic diseases, support mental health, and reduce the risk of heart disease. Seafood, particularly shellfish, is also rich in vitamins like B12, iodine, and zinc, which can boost your immunity and support your thyroid function, both of which can begin to decline the older we get.
- **Avocados:** Not only are avocados creamy and delicious, but they also provide a seemingly endless supply of nutrients. This long list includes potassium, which promotes healthy blood pressure levels. Avocados are also packed with monounsaturated fats that can reduce bad cholesterol levels, potentially lowering the risk of heart disease. Additionally, the fiber in avocados helps with digestion and can give you a feeling of fullness that lasts for hours, reducing your urge to snack during your fasting window.
- **Potatoes:** With a rich supply of vital nutrients like potassium, potatoes play an essential role in heart function and muscle contractions. They also provide a variety of vitamins, including vitamin C, which boosts your immune function and enhances your skin health. Potatoes also contain vitamin B6, which plays a crucial role in brain development and assists with specific enzyme reactions that strengthen your metabolism.

Remember this vital fact - preparation matters; roasted or boiled is always a healthier choice than fried!

- **Green Vegetables:** Leafy greens like spinach are rich in iron, calcium, and essential vitamins like K, A, and C. Kale is chock-full of antioxidants like quercetin and kaempferol and is also one of the world's best sources of Vitamin K. Broccoli is not just high in fiber but also has a decent amount of proteins compared to other vegetables. This vegetable's density can keep you feeling full for an extended period.

- **Whole Grains:** Whole grains, as opposed to refined grains, keep all parts of the grain intact, ensuring a healthy dose of fiber, protein, and essential vitamins and minerals. Quinoa, a complete protein, also contains ample amounts of fiber, magnesium, and phosphorus. Oats are among the healthiest grains on earth and are a great source of essential nutrients and antioxidants. Brown rice is nutrient-rich, especially in fiber, which helps with digestion and keeps you feeling full.

- **Nuts:** Nuts are little bundles of nutrients. Almonds, for instance, are loaded with vitamin E, magnesium, and fiber. Walnuts are full of antioxidants and one of the richest sources of Omega-3 fatty acids. Cashews provide good, healthy fats and are also an excellent protein source. They're also rich in magnesium, beneficial for bone health, and reduce high blood pressure, which is especially important as we age.

- **Fermented Foods:** Many foods undergo a fermentation process that allows for the growth of beneficial bacteria, also known as probiotics. Yogurt provides probiotics and is a good source of calcium and protein. Kimchi, a spicy Korean side dish, is rich in vitamins A and C, and its main ingredient, cabbage, provides ample fiber. Sauerkraut, which is fermented cabbage, boosts your digestive tract's health with its probiotics supply and provides vitamins C, B, and K.

Foods to Avoid

Knowing which foods to cut back on or avoid is just as crucial as knowing which foods to consume while fasting. Let's talk about some of these foods and the reasons why you should stay away from them as much as possible:

- **Sugary Foods:** Sugary foods might be tempting but can quickly raise blood sugar levels. Once these levels drop again, we might feel tired, dizzy, or even a bit grumpy. Plus, they only keep us full for a short time. Over time, consuming too much sugar can lead to weight gain and other health challenges.
- **Processed Foods:** Processed foods can harm and derail our efforts towards good health. Manufacturers often modify these foods from their natural state by adding excessive additives and preservatives. They might lack the nutrients our bodies crave; some added ingredients can make us want to eat even more. They're not the best choice when trying to get the most from our eating window. Our local grocery stores feature processed foods predominantly in the middle aisles and freezer sections.
- **Excessive Caffeine:** A cup of coffee or tea can be lovely to help us get moving in the morning. However, consuming too much caffeine can lead to dehydration and overstimulation. Plus, taking it late in the day might interfere with our sleep. Limit caffeine as much as possible and stick to only one mug daily.
- **Excessive Alcohol:** An occasional glass of wine or beer is one thing, but too much alcohol isn't ideal for anyone

of any age. Alcohol gives us "empty calories," meaning we take in extra calories without getting any valuable nutrients. It can also disrupt our sleep, leaving us tired the next day. It may also have a diuretic effect, causing us to become dehydrated and leaving us more thirsty.

- **Calorie-Dense Treats:** Pastries, donuts, cakes, and similar treats are often loaded with calories and offer little nutrition for our bodies. They can make us feel full and satisfied for a short time, but we usually find ourselves hungry again soon after. These treats are also full of sugar and fat, which can sabotage any weight loss goals that we may be trying to achieve.

WHY IS HEALTHY EATING IMPORTANT?

As we age into our 50s and beyond, we encounter several physiological changes. Most of these changes occur from shifts in our hormone levels. Menopause typically occurs during this period, leading to decreased estrogen levels. This decline can influence different aspects of your health, from bone density to cardiovascular health and even how quickly your metabolism runs. Here are some important facts about your health as you age and why you should make good nutrition a part of your daily routine:

- **Bone Health:** As estrogen levels drop, bone breakdown can outpace bone formation, leading to decreased bone density and a greater risk of fractures. Foods rich in calcium and vitamin D, like fish, dairy, and fermented foods, can help give your body the calcium it needs to promote more vital bone health.
- **Metabolism and Weight Management:** Metabolism tends to slow down with age; if you're anything like me, you are probably already experiencing this. A slower

metabolism, combined with hormonal changes, can lead to weight gain, especially around the midsection. Including metabolism-boosting foods in your diet, like protein-rich eggs and fish, can help maintain muscle mass and promote a healthy metabolic rate. Eating plenty of protein causes the body to work harder during digestion and metabolism, which forces our body to use more energy and, therefore, burn more calories - especially during sleep. On top of this, fueling your body with healthy fats like those in avocados and nuts can aid in weight management by promoting satiety and reducing your overall caloric intake.

- **Cardiovascular Health:** Post-menopause, there's a significant increase in the risk of cardiovascular diseases for women. Omega-3 fatty acids, found in fish and nuts, are proven to reduce blood pressure and prevent the buildup of harmful plaque in the arteries. Potassium, found in foods like avocados and potatoes, also plays a role in maintaining healthy blood pressure.
- **Digestive Health:** The digestive system slows with age, leading to pesky issues like constipation. The fiber found in whole grains, green vegetables, and avocados can help with smoother digestion and promote a healthy gut. With their probiotics, fermented foods support a balanced gut microbiome, further ensuring good digestive health.
- **Skin and Hair Health:** Nutrient deficiencies can reflect on your skin and hair. Poor eating habits can lead to hair loss, dry, brittle hair, and a dull complexion. The antioxidants in green vegetables, the biotin in eggs, and the healthy fats in avocados and nuts can help give you the radiant skin and healthy hair you deserve!
- **Cognitive Health:** Omega-3 fatty acids, found abundantly in fish, play a role in keeping your brain

healthy and functioning with clarity. These foods can protect against age-related cognitive decline and reduce the risk of degenerative diseases like dementia and Alzheimer's Disease.

When you mix intermittent fasting with a healthy diet filled with power-packed foods, you get the best of both worlds. While fasting helps repair cells, control blood sugar, and burn fat, the good foods you eat give your body the extra boost it needs, especially as you age. So, for women over 50, these foods will help you meet your specific nutritional needs and allow you to get the most out of your intermittent fasting regimen.

STAYING HYDRATED: THE ROLE OF H2O

Hydration is essential for good health. For women over 50, maintaining proper hydration levels is one of the most important things you can do to support your body's changing needs. Intermittent fasting poses a unique challenge in this regard. With a limited eating window each day, there's a risk that you may drink less than you normally would. While the focus of IF is usually on food, paying attention to the importance of drinking plenty of fluids and staying hydrated is essential.

Water isn't just something to quench our thirst. It plays many vital roles in our bodies. It helps digest our food, ensuring we can properly absorb the necessary nutrients. For women over 50, proper hydration also plays a crucial role in the health of our skin. It has the ability to maintain our skin's hydration, giving it a fresh and vibrant look. Water does more than hydrate the skin; it's also essential for the brain. It helps us with concentration, memory, and mood, all things that become even more essential as we age.

On top of all this, intermittent fasting puts the body into a state where it's busy with processes like cellular repair and fat burning. These processes require energy and the right environment to be efficient. Without proper hydration, the body can't perform these tasks to the best of its ability. Think of water as your body's support crew, ensuring everything flows smoothly, especially during IF. For women over 50 practicing intermittent fasting, staying hydrated throughout the day can be an absolute game-changer and will help you feel your very best.

What to Drink

While water remains the top choice, there are several other beverages that you can enjoy for both their taste and health benefits, which will quench your thirst and help keep you hydrated. Each of these drinks offers its own set of advantages, ensuring you have plenty of options to choose from.

- **Water:** This is our body's primary hydration source. It's calorie-free, helps flush out toxins, and supports almost every body function. Frequent daily water intake is the simplest and most effective way to stay hydrated. Whenever possible, choose filtered water to ensure that you are getting the purest form possible.
- **Herbal Teas:** Herbal teas are calorie-free drinks that hydrate and offer many other benefits depending on your chosen type. For instance, chamomile can be soothing and help with sleep, while peppermint can be invigorating and help improve digestion. With its fat-burning properties, green tea can help improve metabolism, and the caffeine it packs can perk up your mind and body. Drinking herbal teas can also provide warmth and comfort, especially during colder days.

- **Bone Broth:** Bone broth isn't just a drink. It can be like a light, nourishing meal in a cup. It's packed with essential minerals like calcium and magnesium, and for women over 50, these nutrients can be especially beneficial, supporting your bone health and overall well-being. It also has a savory flavor that can be satisfying during fasting hours, helping you overcome any hunger pangs you may be experiencing.
- **Coffee:** A favorite for many, coffee in moderation can give you an energy boost and is a great way to start your day. It's rich in antioxidants, which are vital for overall health. If you choose to have coffee during your fasting window, it's best to have it black or with minimal cream to ensure it doesn't break your fast. It is also best to drink coffee in moderation as its diuretic effects can cause you to become dehydrated, and too much caffeine can make you feel jittery.
- **Unsweetened Almond Milk and Coconut Water:** These drinks can be a great choice if you are tired of plain water. Almond milk, when unsweetened, is low in calories and can be a source of calcium and vitamin E. Coconut water is very hydrating. It can provide essential electrolytes like potassium, making it a good choice, especially after a workout.

TIPS TO STAY ON TRACK WITH PROPER NUTRITION

As with anything we do, one of the best ways to ensure success is to be prepared. Making the right food and drink choices can maximize the benefits of IF, ensuring you feel your best and stay energized. To help navigate this journey with ease, here are some practical tips to keep your eating and drinking habits on track:

- **Set Clear Goals:** Understand why you're doing IF. Whether it's for weight loss, improved energy, or better health, keep this goal in mind.
- **Plan Your Eating Window:** Choose a consistent time frame that fits your lifestyle and stick to it.
- **Stay Hydrated:** Drink plenty of water throughout the day, especially during fasting hours.
- **Prepare Nutrient-Dense Meals:** Focus on whole foods rich in vitamins, minerals, and fiber.
- **Avoid Empty Calories:** Skip sugary or processed foods that offer little nutritional value.
- **Limit Caffeine:** One or two cups of coffee are okay, but excessive caffeine can disrupt sleep.
- **Opt for Herbal Teas:** These can be hydrating and offer additional health benefits.
- **Practice Mindful Eating:** Listen to your hunger cues and savor each bite.
- **Start with a Balanced Meal:** Ensure your first meal post-fasting has protein, healthy fats, and fiber.
- **Avoid Overeating:** Eating a lot after a fast can be tempting, but listen to your body and stop when you're full.
- **Limit Alcohol:** Alcohol can dehydrate and interfere with the benefits of IF.
- **Keep Healthy Snacks On Hand:** For moments when you need something quick, have options like nuts or fruit available.
- **Stay Active:** Light exercises during fasting can be beneficial and can help keep your mind off of food.
- **Get Plenty of Sleep:** Restful sleep can aid recovery and reduce hunger pangs.
- **Avoid Sugary Drinks:** Stick to water, herbal teas, or unsweetened beverages.

- **Educate Yourself:** The more you know about IF and good nutrition, the better choices you can make.
- **Be Flexible:** If something isn't working, adjust your approach. IF should fit your life, not the other way around. This also goes for the foods you eat. If you don't like something, replace it with another healthy choice that you enjoy.
- **Stay Connected:** Join online groups or forums to share experiences, gain support, and share recipes and nutrition tips.
- **Listen to Your Body:** If you feel unwell or overly tired, consider adjusting your fasting window, changing your meals, or speaking to a nutritionist or physician.
- **Stay Consistent:** Like any other habit, consistency is key. Stick to your routine and make adjustments as needed.
- **Be Prepared:** Ensure your fridge and pantry are filled with healthy and nutritious choices. Prepping your meals and snacks ahead of time will ensure that you always have something healthy to eat when hunger strikes.

My Journey with Nutrition

I used to find myself grabbing a pastry for breakfast and stopping at a nearby cafeteria or fast food joint for lunch. By the time I made it through the door in the evenings, dinner was a phone call away to the nearest pizza delivery place. Food was about comfort and convenience when I was growing up. I never stopped to think about the nutritional value of my eating. But as I approached my 50s, I started seeing and feeling the consequences of my food choices, and I knew something had to change.

When I decided to start intermittent fasting, I wanted to make sure that I gave my body the best chance possible for success. I took a proactive approach. I began planning my meals each week. Every Sunday, armed with my list, I'd go grocery shopping. I focused on fresh vegetables, lean proteins, and healthy fats. I discovered the joy of cooking meals at home, exploring new recipes, and controlling what went into my body.

Meal prepping became my secret weapon. I'd set aside a few hours each week to prepare meals and snacks. This simple act transformed my eating habits. I no longer reached for unhealthy choices out of convenience; I had nutritious meals ready whenever I needed them.

Over time, I felt better. My energy levels increased, my skin looked brighter, and I felt more in tune with my body's needs. I also stopped craving unhealthy foods and found myself reaching for healthy snacks, like fruits and veggies. Proper grocery shopping and meal prep were my game-changers. It's never too late to make positive changes, and for me, understanding and respecting nutrition was the first step towards a healthier, happier me.

Moving Forward

This chapter has been about the world of nutrition and how it plays a decisive role in our lives, especially as we enter our 50s and beyond. While understanding what to eat is essential, knowing how it pairs with other aspects of our well-being can help us maximize our health journey even more.

So, what's up next? We will get moving and discover how to combine training and exercise with intermittent fasting successfully. For many women over 50, the thought of merging these two might feel challenging, but don't worry. We will look at how to strike the right balance, ensuring you get the most out of your exercise and fasting routine without feeling overwhelmed or exhausted. We will explore how to tailor workouts to your body's unique needs and ensure that your physical activity matches perfectly with your fasting schedule. Doing so will enhance your weight loss, fire up your metabolism, and boost your health!

6

T: TRAINING AND EXERCISE WHILE FASTING

 "Take care of your body. It's the only place you have to live."

— JIM ROHN

These words mean a lot to me and represent a way of living I have tried to embrace my entire life. I've always loved staying active, but I also knew that fasting would change how much energy my body would use. I was excited to change my dietary habits and find a new way to fuel my body. However, as a fitness enthusiast, I wondered, "Could I go for hours without eating and still have the energy to stay active and get in the workouts that I love?"

Fortunately, the answer is a resounding yes!

IF gives us the opportunity to understand the body's unique rhythms better, allowing us to be even more in tune with ourselves and how we feel. It can also be a great energy booster. It gave me a push far greater than anything I had experienced in years!

In the pages that follow, we are going to take a look at how IF and exercise can work together. How we can easily find the energy we need to wake up alert and get through our daily activities (including a workout routine!) with ease.

EXERCISE TIPS WHILE FASTING

While exercise and intermittent fasting go hand-in-hand for your overall health, you may experience some ups and downs, especially in the beginning. Knowing which speed bumps to watch out for and how to handle them when they arise can make this journey much easier and more successful.

The Pros and Cons of Exercising While Fasting

It's not uncommon for many people to have their reservations about exercising while fasting. This is a normal feeling and many of us might wonder if it's really a good mix. Here's a quick breakdown of what I've experienced and learned:

✛ Pros:

- **Enhanced Fat Burn:** On an empty stomach, the body taps into fat reserves for energy, which can help boost the body's ability to burn fat.
- **Mental Clarity:** By fasting, you can rejuvenate your morning fitness routines and maintain keen awareness throughout the day.
- **Improved Metabolism:** Exercising in a fasted state can ramp up metabolism, helping you reach your weight loss goals faster and increasing your body's fat-burning potential throughout the day.

— Cons:

- **Reduced Energy:** Initially, you might feel a dip in stamina without your usual pre-workout meal.
- **Muscle Stress:** You can lose muscle if you exercise too hard and don't refuel your body properly afterward.
- **Possible Dizziness:** Fasting and exercising can lead to dizziness for some people. This issue can often be avoided by easing into workouts, listening to your body, and staying hydrated.

How to Work Out Safely and Efficiently While Practicing IF

I remember my first workout while fasting. I was nervous and excited all at the same time. I noticed a definite decrease in my energy levels and couldn't push myself as hard as usual. At the same time, I was hopeful to see better results than I normally would expect in the gym. Getting in a good caloric burn, combined with my fasted state, would help me burn fat faster. By following these tips, I was able to get the most out of my workouts and boosted my energy levels over time while ensuring that I stayed safe:

- **Stay Hydrated:** Drink plenty of water before and after your workout to prevent dehydration.
- **Listen to Your Body:** If you feel too drained or dizzy, it's okay to take a break and start again later.
- **Start Slow:** If you're new to fasted workouts, begin with low-impact exercises and gradually increase the intensity.
- **Optimal Timing:** Many find it easier to work out towards the end of their fasting window, right before their first meal. You can also choose to work out later in the day, not in a fasted state.

- **Nutrition is Key:** After exercising, eat a balanced meal with proteins, healthy fats, and carbs to speed up recovery.
- **Stay Consistent:** It's better to stick to moderate exercises regularly than to push too hard on certain days and feel drained on others.
- **Warm-up Properly:** A good warm-up prepares your body, especially when working out on an empty stomach.
- **Focus on Form:** It's easy to rush through exercises. Instead, take your time and concentrate on getting your form right to prevent injuries.
- **Stay Flexible:** There were days when I felt more energetic than others. It's okay to adjust your routine based on how you feel. Take a day off if needed, or choose lower-impact activities that align with how your body is feeling.

Syncing Your Exercise with Your Fasting Schedule

Finding the sweet spot between fasting and exercising can take some trial and error, but the results will speak for themselves once you find the right rhythm. Balancing both exercise and fasting can maximize your health and weight loss benefits, and here are the best ways to go about managing it:

- **Time It Right:** Consider exercising a couple of hours before you break your fast. This timing allows you to finish your workout and then indulge in a nutrient-rich meal to help boost your recovery.
- **Adjust Intensity:** Some days, you might feel lighter and more agile, making brisk walks or light cardio a great choice. When you feel extra energized, consider strength training or more intensive exercises. If you are

feeling sluggish or lethargic, opt for easy stretches or take a rest day.

- **Plan Meals Around Workouts:** If you are getting in a strenuous workout, plan your meal times properly. Ensure you eat right afterward to start recovery and fuel your body with healthy proteins and good carbs for maximum results.
- **Rest Is Important:** Combining fasting with exercise can be demanding on your body. Ensure you're giving your body the rest it needs. Prioritizing quality sleep and routinely adding rest days to your schedule is essential.

The idea is to create harmony and balance between fasting and exercising. Remember, it's about complementing, not competing. Each body is unique, so finding what works best for you is essential. Remember, the goal is to feel good and take a step towards a healthier you each day. Even baby steps are steps in the right direction!

CREATING YOUR PERFECT EXERCISE ROUTINE

Starting a new health journey is exciting, right? It's about committing to yourself and your well-being and overcoming the challenges you may face head-on. If you're anything like me, you have seen your share of good and bad days, meaning you are probably an expert at taking what life throws at you and just going with the flow. Sometimes, however, we all need a little bit of guidance. Creating the perfect exercise routine can be overwhelming. It can take time to figure out where to start. t. Fortunately, I have some tips and tricks to help you create a plan to help you meet your health goals and stay in line with all the impressive goals you aim to achieve.

Your Step-by-Step Guide to Fitness Planning

1. Assess Your Current State:

Before diving into any routine, knowing where you stand is crucial. Consider any health conditions, your current fitness level, and how active you've been lately. Understanding these can help you set realistic goals that are safe for your body. It is also a good idea to consult with your family physician. They can tell you what activities suit you best based on your current health status.

2. Identify Your Goals:

What do you want to achieve? Whether it's weight loss, muscle strength, increased flexibility, or improved heart health, being clear on your primary goals can help you make the right exercise choices.

3. Choose Activities You Enjoy:

Exercise shouldn't be a chore. Select activities you love. Try new things like dancing, swimming or cycling and find the one that fits best with your lifestyle. You're more likely to stick to it when you enjoy it.

4. Incorporate Variety:

Your body thrives on diversity. A mix of cardio, strength training, and flexibility exercises ensures a well-rounded routine. By mixing it up, you will increase fat burn, improve balance and flexibility, and experience muscle gains.

5. Schedule and Consistency:

Plan your workouts around your fasting windows. Find a time of day that feels best for you and stick with it. Consistency is crucial when it comes to seeing results. While adjusting your routine based on how you feel is okay, stick with it and stay motivated.

6. Adjust and Adapt:

As you work out, your body will change, and so will your stamina levels. Take time every few weeks to regularly review and tweak your plan based on your progress and feelings.

Building Your Routine

Here are the nine most important steps to help you shape an exercise routine that fits perfectly into your life. By following these tips, you can ensure optimal results and a routine to stick to. Let's get started!

Step #1: Determine your "Get in Shape" situation!

Start by assessing your current fitness level. Are you active or mostly sedentary? What physical activities do you enjoy? Knowing your starting point helps you pick suitable exercises. Understanding where you stand is critical whether you're beginning a new exercise regimen or returning after a break. This self-awareness enables you to set achievable goals and ensures that your journey is rewarding and tailored perfectly for you.

Step #2: What exercises should I do to lose weight (or build muscle)?

Choosing the right exercises depends on your goals. If you want to lose weight, focus on a mix of cardio exercises like walking or swimming. These help burn more calories and boost heart health. If building muscle is your goal, include strength training exercises using weights or resistance bands. Everyone's body is different, so finding what you enjoy and what feels good for you is essential.

Step #3: How many sets and reps should I do per exercise?

When starting, it's good to aim for 2-3 sets of 10-15 repetitions for each exercise. This range is effective for strength building and can boost your endurance. You can adjust the sets and reps according to your goals as you get stronger. Remember, listening to your body is crucial; if you feel pain or discomfort, lower your reps or take a break. Always make sure you are prioritizing safety.

Step #4: Resting Between Sets

After completing a set, allow yourself a short break before moving to the next. For strength exercises, waiting 60-90 seconds is the perfect amount of time. This rest allows your muscles to recover, will enable you to catch your breath, and prepares you for the next set.

Step #5: How do I choose the proper weight?

Start with a weight that feels manageable but slightly challenging. As a guideline, the last two reps of your set should be challenging but doable. If it's too easy, add a little weight. If it's too hard, there's no shame in reducing it.

Step #6: How long should I exercise for?

Aim for a 30-minute workout when starting. If 30 minutes feels too harsh, break it into shorter 10-minute segments. Over time, as your stamina improves, you can gradually increase the duration. Remember, consistency is more valuable than intensity. It's about creating a routine that suits your lifestyle and is sustainable.

Step #7: Incorporating Supersets and Circuit Training

Supersets involve doing two exercises back-to-back with no rest in between. For example, you might do a set of squats followed immediately by push-ups. Circuit training is a series of exercises done in sequence, often targeting different muscle groups. You might do a round of squats, push-ups, and jumping jacks in a circuit. Both methods can maximize your workout and are especially good when pressed for time.

Step #8: How often should I train?

Training 3-4 days a week is a good start for most people. It provides recovery days in between, which are just as important as workout days. Remember, it's not about how often you train but how consistent you are. Find a schedule that aligns with your lifestyle and make it your goal to stick to it.

Step #9: How to Track Your Progress

If you have stayed on top of the latest trends, you have probably found yourself writing in a journal once or twice. Whether you have kept a food journal, an affirmations journal, or a gratitude journal, you have likely seen their benefits. Keeping a workout journal is an excellent way to track your progress. It can also help motivate you, giving you the determination to push forward. When you write in your journal, keep track of your exercises, the number of sets and reps you perform, and how much weight you lift. Over time, you will be able to see the improvements in your strength and endurance levels. Alternatively, many fitness apps can help you track your workouts digitally if you are tech-savvy. Alternatively, many fitness apps can help you track your workouts digitally if you are tech-savvy.

SAMPLE WORKOUT PLAN FOR BEGINNERS

Every journey starts with a single step! If you are hesitant about starting a new routine, don't worry - you're not alone! Most women can feel apprehensive about exercise. Maybe we don't know what to do, where to start, or how to perform a particular exercise. Fortunately, the good thing about exercise is you just have to keep moving! As time passes, you will become more confident and ready to try new things. For now, we have created this easy workout plan for beginners. Start here, stick to it, and when you are comfortable, you can make changes that fit with your lifestyle and goals.

Monday: Low-Impact Cardio

Warm-up: 5-minute brisk walk

Main Activity: 20-minute walk, steadily increasing your pace.

Cool down: 5-minute slow walk and gentle stretching

Tuesday: Strength Training (Upper Body)

Warm-up: Arm circles

Main Activity:

- Dumbbell bicep curls: 3 sets of 12 reps
- Overhead tricep extensions: 3 sets of 12 reps
- Dumbbell shoulder press: 3 sets of 12 reps

Cool down: Stretch arms and shoulders for 5 minutes

Wednesday: Rest or Short Walk

Thursday: Strength Training (Lower Body)

Warm-up: Standing Leg Circles

Main Activity:

- Bodyweight squats: 3 sets of 15 reps
- Walking Lunges: 3 sets of 15 reps on each leg
- Glute bridges: 2 sets of 15 reps

Cool down: Stretch legs and lower back for 5 minutes

Friday: Low-Impact Cardio

Warm-up: 5-minute brisk walk

Main Activity: 20-minute walk, switching between an average and brisk pace every 2 minutes.

Cool down: 5-minute slow walk and gentle stretching

Saturday: Active Recovery

Try out any light activity you enjoy: dancing, gardening, or a leisurely bike ride are perfect choices. This active recovery day keeps your muscles moving without being too strenuous.

Sunday: Rest and Reflect

This plan offers the perfect mix of cardiovascular exercises and strength training. It was made with women like us in mind to help boost our endurance and increase our muscle mass. Remember, it's vital to remain aware of your body's feedback and adjust the intensity as required. As your fitness skills advance, you should increase your reps and sets or extend the duration of each session. Prioritize steady progress over perfection, and approach each stage of your fitness journey with dedication towards continued improvement.

Other Exercises You Can Try

- **Swimming:** Provides resistance for muscle strength while being easy on the joints.
- **Tai Chi:** Enhances balance, flexibility, and mental well-being.
- **Pilates:** Strengthens the core, improves posture, and boosts flexibility.
- **Water Aerobics:** Cardio exercise that uses water resistance to minimize joint stress.
- **Resistance Band Exercises:** Build strength without the need for heavy weights.
- **Cycling:** Using a stationary bike can be a great low-impact cardio option.
- **Elliptical Trainer:** Provides a full-body workout without the hard impact of running.
- **Dance:** Classes like ballroom or line dancing can be fun and physically beneficial.
- **Chair Exercises:** Ideal for those with mobility issues or when standing is challenging.
- **Golf:** Walking the course provides exercise, and swinging helps with flexibility.
- **Bowling:** Great for socializing while also moving and engaging the muscles.
- **Stretching:** Daily routines can help maintain flexibility and reduce stiffness.
- **Balance Exercises:** Stand on one foot, heel-to-toe walk, or leg lifts can improve stability.

Finding my Rhythm

At 52, life took a different turn for me. My house was quieter with my kids grown, and I felt an urge for something new. That's when I considered upping my exercise game while continuing intermittent fasting. I wondered, "Can I actually do more physical activity without compromising my health?"

The first few days were challenging. I was experiencing significant dips in my energy. Working out was a challenge, and I felt tired throughout the day. But I didn't want to give up. Instead, I changed my approach. I started my days with gentle stretching sessions during the fasting period. It was a simple, peaceful way to wake up my body.

Things clicked when I introduced light cardio in the afternoons, right before my main meal. Taking a brisk walk or bike ride through my neighborhood became my daily routine. This timing was a game-changer. Post-exercise, I could refuel my body with a healthy meal, giving my body the fuel it needed for proper recovery.

Once I got more comfortable, I felt bold enough to include resistance training several times a week. It was surprising how, on some days, I'd wake up feeling more energetic than usual. On those days, I'd challenge myself more, add a few more reps, or increase my walking pace. It was essential for me to listen to my body and do what felt right on that specific day.

I am proud to say that my results were nothing short of astonishing. Not only did I drop a few stubborn pounds, but my stamina improved. My skin had a post-workout glow that even my friends and family noticed. More than the physical benefits, though, was this feeling of achieving something big. I learned that my body could adapt in ways I hadn't imagined.

This experience taught me a lot. It wasn't just about fitness or weight loss. It was about paying attention to my body's signals and finding what worked for me. With IF and exercise, I established a routine that wasn't burdensome but became a natural part of my life.

Fitness and Fasting - Tying it All Together

Throughout this chapter, we've talked about the nuances of fitness and how to combine this with your IF journey. You've learned the importance of creating a personalized workout plan, got insights on reps and sets, and the importance of including proper rest in your routine. Remember, proper training, motivation, and dedication can work wonders regardless of age.

The next chapter of this book will cover the W in FASTWISE: Well-Being and the Challenges You May Face during your intermittent fasting journey. Many women over 50 encounter unique challenges while practicing intermittent fasting. We'll address concerns like adjusting to social gatherings, handling family meals, and staying motivated - even during the most challenging times. Awareness of these issues will fuel you to face them head-on and keep pushing toward your health goals. Stick with us, and let's conquer these challenges together!

7

W: WELL-BEING AND THE CHALLENGES YOU MAY FACE

> "On fasting days, picture your ideal body and remember that your body is dipping into its fat reserve for energy and repairing damaged cells. Let that knowledge encourage and support you. Feel your food addiction weakening its hold on you."
>
> — DAVID ORTNER

Starting intermittent fasting might sound simple: you eat during specific hours and fast during the rest. But, like any significant lifestyle change, it can come with unexpected challenges. If you're anything like I was, you may have noticed that some days are harder than others or wondered why certain symptoms appear unexpectedly. It's completely normal to hit a few road bumps along the way - this happens to the best of us! In this next part of our journey, we will look at some of the common issues women face with intermittent fasting, and I will give you all the tools you need to overcome them. Let's address these challenges and find solutions together!

DEALING WITH FOOD SENSITIVITIES

Did you know that Intermittent fasting might change how your body reacts to certain foods? Some people notice that their food sensitivities reduce over time. These food sensitivities happen because fasting gives your digestive system a much-needed break, which can help ease any inflammation it may be experiencing. You might see improvements if you have previously felt bloated or got a rash after eating certain foods. However, it's important to introduce foods slowly and watch how your body responds. If you've had severe allergic reactions in the past, always consult a doctor before making changes. Remember, intermittent fasting isn't just about when you eat but also about understanding and listening to your body's unique needs.

Environmental Toxins

When you practice intermittent fasting, your body works extra hard to cleanse itself, including tackling environmental toxins. These toxins can come from everyday sources like processed foods, air pollution, and household products. When fasting, your body might release stored toxins as it burns fat for energy. You could feel off during this detox process. To give your body extra support during this time, consider eating organic foods, using natural household products, and drinking plenty of water to help flush things out faster. Also, by being mindful of the toxins you expose yourself to daily, you can enhance the cleansing benefits of your fasting routine.

Handling Hidden Infections

Sometimes, our bodies can suffer from minor, hidden infections we aren't aware of. These infections can sometimes impact how you feel during your fasting periods. These infections might not always show apparent symptoms but can affect your energy levels and overall well-being. If you've started fasting and suddenly feel more tired or unwell, your body could be dealing with these underlying issues. Remember to consult with a healthcare professional if you suspect an infection or are unsure about any changes in your health.

Nutritional Deficiencies

While intermittent fasting can offer many benefits, it's imperative to ensure you're still getting all the nutrients your body needs on a daily basis. Skipping meals might lead to missing out on vital vitamins and minerals. It's not just about eating less but ensuring that when you do eat, you are eating right. Prioritize nutrient-dense foods, like leafy greens, lean proteins, and whole grains, during your eating window. Supplements can be an option, but always consult a nutritionist or doctor before adding them to your routine. Remember, the goal is to boost your health, and that means making sure every meal counts towards meeting your specific nutritional needs.

Feeling Sick or Lethargic

If you're feeling a bit off or tired during fasting, you're not alone. As your body adjusts to a new eating pattern, it's prevalent for women to experience some fatigue or sluggishness. Think of it as your system resetting itself. To overcome this, make sure you're drinking plenty of water, and when you do eat, select balanced meals that provide enough fuel for your body. Also, permit yourself to rest more if needed. As always, listen to your body's signals. If these feelings persist or feel severe, talking with a health professional might be a good idea to ensure fasting is right for you.

Coping with Rapid Weight Loss

Have you noticed you're shedding pounds a bit too quickly while fasting? For some, especially as we age, losing weight too fast can be a significant concern. Rapid weight loss can sometimes lead to loss of muscle mass and reduced bone density. Focus on consuming nutrient-rich foods during your eating windows to ensure you're losing weight slowly and steadily. For instance, protein and calcium (from dairy sources) can support muscle and bone health. You can also increase your caloric intake during your eating window or reduce your fasting times to ensure you have enough time to get all the food your body requires without burning it off too quickly.

MANAGING MEDICATIONS

If you're taking medications, it's important to consider how they could interact with your fasting routine. Some medicines require food for proper absorption, while others might cause side effects on an empty stomach. Also, certain medications can affect blood sugar levels, making fasting more challenging. Before starting any new lifestyle changes, take some time to chat with your doctor or pharmacist. They are the experts about medication and will be able to provide knowledgeable insight on the best timing for your medications with your fasting window. They might recommend adjusting your dosage or suggest an alternative medication more compatible with fasting. Always remember: your health and safety come first. While fasting has many benefits, ensuring that your prescriptions work effectively and safely is the primary focus.

MANAGING SOCIAL AND FAMILY LIFE

Having an active social life is very important, especially as we age. However, social gatherings while fasting can be tricky to maneuver. However, they are entirely possible with some planning and can still be fun! Fasting should allow you to enjoy time with loved ones or attend special events. With the right approach, you can balance your fasting goals with the joys of socializing. Here's how:

Tips for Integrating Fasting into Your Social Life

- **Open Communication:** Let friends and family know about your fasting routine. Their understanding can give you the support you need.
- **Plan Ahead:** When attending social events, check the menu beforehand. Adjust your eating window if necessary, or choose foods that align with your fasting and health goals.
- **Stay Hydrated:** Opt for water or herbal teas if the event occurs within your fasting window. This way, you're still a part of the party without having to break your fast.
- **Focus on Social Interactions:** Remember, gatherings are just as much about the company as they are about the food. Cherish the conversations and the time you spend with those close to you.
- **Give Yourself Grace:** If you make an exception for a special occasion, it's okay. Enjoy your time, and get back on track the next day. It's important to allow yourself these breaks to enjoy your life as well. You shouldn't feel guilty about it!

Enjoying Meals With Loved Ones While Staying On Track

Navigating meals with family and friends while staying on track with your fasting goals can be delicate to balance. But, with a little mindfulness, you can savor those shared moments without deviating too far from your plan. Here's how:

- **Mindful Eating:** Truly savor each bite. This not only enhances enjoyment but can also help you recognize when you're full.
- **Portion Control:** Choose smaller plates. You'll likely eat less but still feel satisfied, especially during gatherings where you expect food to be abundant.
- **Prioritize Protein and Veggies:** Fill most of your plate with protein and veggies. Loading up on these provides the necessary nutrients without the risk of indulging too much in unhealthy options.
- **Limit Distractions:** Engaging wholeheartedly in discussions and minimizing phone distractions ensures you savor the present moment, enjoy social interactions, and become more attuned to your body's signals.

Handling challenges of intermittent fasting in various social scenarios

There are many different social scenarios that you may encounter during your IF journey. Being prepared for these situations ahead of time can help you handle them in a way that best aligns with your health and wellness goals.

- **Periods of Fasting:** When fasting coincides with a social event, you might feel out of sync. It is important to remember in this situation that you're in control. If you're not eating, engage in conversations and enjoy the company. It's okay to explain you're fasting, but don't feel obligated to justify your choices to anyone.

- **IF Goes to a Restaurant:** Eating out doesn't mean breaking your fast prematurely. Look at the menu beforehand, choose something that fits your eating window or preferences, and enjoy it. If it's not your eating time, opt for a calorie-free beverage and savor the moment instead.
- **Having Fun while Dining Out:** Fasting shouldn't sideline your fun. Engage in the ambiance, enjoy your drink (even if it's just water with lemon), and immerse yourself in the company and conversation that is taking place around you. Remember, the joy should come from the experience, not just the food.
- **IF's Family Get-Togethers:** Family gatherings can be tricky when fasting. It is important to remember that these times should focus on togetherness, not just the food.
- **Strategies for Enjoying Gatherings:** When attending events, focus on the joy of socializing. Bring a fasting-friendly snack, or plan your eating window around the event. Celebrate the moments, not just the meals.
- **Societal Constraints and IF:** Society often revolves around meals. When faced with questions or misunderstandings about your fasting lifestyle, be patient. Educate the people around you on your choice if asked, but also know it's okay to state your personal choices without having to elaborate or justify them.
- **Managing Stress while Fasting:** Stress can tempt you to break your fast. Find a deeper sense of calm with deep breathing exercises, a walk, or a short meditation session. When stressful situations creep up, remember why you started this journey and let that guide you through the stressful times.

STAYING MOTIVATED

Staying motivated, especially during a transformative journey like intermittent fasting, is vital. There were many times that I had to dig deep and give it my all to stick with it. Think of motivation as the fuel for your journey. Without it, it's easy to stall or veer entirely off track. For many women, IF isn't just about weight loss or a healthier lifestyle. Many women are attracted to this way of eating because it challenges them to step outside of their comfort zone and push their boundaries to the limit. But, as with all changes, there can be moments of doubt - I know I've had my share of them! Next up are some ways to keep that motivational fire burning brightly and ensure you stay committed and enjoy all the fantastic benefits that come along with your efforts.

Overcoming challenges and staying focused – Techniques to boost self-discipline and commitment

Everyone faces challenges, but it's how you tackle them that counts. When intermittent fasting presents its hurdles, remember why you started. A technique that many find useful is setting clear, achievable milestones instead of vague goals. Celebrate small wins—it can be as simple as sticking to your fasting window for a week straight. Daily affirmations can also keep your mindset positive. Remind yourself, "I am capable," or "Every day, I'm making progress." And don't forget to lean on your support system, whether it's a close friend or an online community. Sharing all parts of your journey, even the ups and the downs can give you a ton of encouragement and some fresh perspectives. Lastly, be kind to yourself. Everyone has off days; they're a part of the process. Recognize them, learn from them, and continue forward with renewed focus.

Ways to Stay Motivated when Doing Intermittent Fasting

Here are some strategies tailored just for you to ensure you stay inspired and determined on this journey.

- **Define goals, not tasks.** Setting clear goals, like achieving better health, is more inspiring than just listing tasks. It gives more purpose to your actions.
- **Move.** Physical activity can elevate your mood and help you feel accomplished. It doesn't have to be intense—a brisk walk, a dance around the kitchen, or some gentle stretching can work wonders - for both your body and your mood!
- **Change your focus.** If you hit a plateau or face a setback, don't dwell on it. Instead, reflect on the progress you've already made and how far you've come, then continue to move forward.
- **Take care of your body.** Listen to what it needs. Stay hydrated, get adequate rest, and eat nutrient-rich foods during your eating windows.
- **Find your deeper why.** Beyond weight loss or health, discover the deeper reason you're fasting. You may be doing this to enjoy playing with your grandchildren, travel the world easily, or embrace a longer, healthier life. Let this 'why' be your anchor and the guiding star that motivates you to keep trying and pushing forward.
- **Focus on positive benefits.** Every time you fast, remember the benefits you're gaining. Think clearer skin, better digestion, and increased energy. These positive outcomes can fuel your motivation.
- **Visualize better health.** Close your eyes and imagine a healthier, more vibrant version of yourself. Visualizing this can make your goals more tangible and achievable.

- **Keep a gratitude journal.** Jot down one thing you're thankful for related to fasting each day. It could be the newfound energy or the discipline you're cultivating. This simple act can shift your mindset and help you think more positively.
- **Fast with a friend.** Sharing the journey makes it more enjoyable. Having someone to discuss experiences with can be a game-changer. Plus, you'll have a buddy to keep you accountable.
- **Reward yourself.** Have you achieved a fasting milestone? Now's the time to celebrate it! Maybe treat yourself to a spa day, a new book, or even a special meal. Reward yourself for all the hard work you've put in and everything you've accomplished.

My Story of Motivation

I won't lie. When I first started intermittent fasting, there were days when I questioned my decision. The initial hunger pangs, adjusting my schedule, and the strange glances from friends as I skipped breakfast were all challenges I faced head-on.

But here's a moment that shifted everything for me. One evening, while on a break from fasting, I was walking by a mirror, and I paused. The reflection I saw was of a woman re-energized and much more vibrant. My skin was clearer, and my eyes looked brighter. That image became my mental anchor.

While the physical changes were significant, the level of mental clarity I experienced was terrific - it had been years since I had felt so alert and focused. My focus sharpened, and my energy levels surged. These transformations became my daily motivators. Every time I felt a hint of doubt, I thought back to that evening and the realization that I had come to.

I began to chat with others, sharing my experiences and listening to theirs. What I realized was that my story had the power to motivate. Just like I drew strength from my own changes, others found encouragement in my journey.

Now, when I think back, it wasn't just about skipping meals or adjusting to a new routine. It was about resilience, determination, and discovering a strength I didn't know I had. I hope my story serves as a reminder to you that challenges are just stepping stones. Each one you overcome brings you closer to your goal. Stay the course, and always remember your 'why'. Remember the reason you started this journey in the first place. Your health, strength, and happiness are going to thank you! Remember that you are worth the effort!

Moving on with Confidence

As we close this chapter, let's take a moment to reflect on what we've learned together. Intermittent fasting is more than just an eating pattern; it's a commitment you make to yourself for a healthier tomorrow. By now, you've got the tools in your arsenal to navigate challenges, whether managing family dinners, staying motivated, or understanding how your body may react to this new lifestyle. Intermittent fasting isn't without its hurdles, but with the nuggets of knowledge I've provided and a dash of determination, you're ready to seize its full potential.

As we move forward, our next chapter dives into the heart of it all: Integrity. We'll explore how staying true to ourselves enhances our journey with intermittent fasting and ensures long-term success. Join me as we continue our path towards better overall wellness, with integrity leading the way.

8

I: INTEGRITY AND LONG-TERM SUCCESS WITH IF

> *"Fasting is the single greatest natural healing therapy. It is nature's ancient, universal 'remedy' for many problems."*
>
> — ELSON HAAS, M.D.

The great thing about IF is its ability to flex with you. Everyone's life, schedule, and body are different. That's why IF is designed to flex with you. Whether you're an early riser or a night owl and have a busy or relaxing day, you can mold a plan that fits your schedule perfectly.

ACCOMMODATING CHANGING NEEDS IN IF SCHEDULES

Life is constantly changing, and so do our routines. As you journey with intermittent fasting, it's okay if your schedule needs some adjustments. Remember, it's about what works best for you. Here are some tips to make sure that IF is always working with you and not against you:

- **Listen to Your Body:** If you feel too hungry or weak during your fasting hours, consider shifting your window. A later start or an earlier end time would feel better.
- **Check Your Calendar:** Have a special breakfast planned? Or a late-night dinner? Adjust your fasting hours for that day. It's okay to make exceptions for special occasions.
- **Ease Into Changes:** If you decide to adjust, make small changes over a few days. For instance, if you want to extend your fasting window, gradually add 30 minutes every few days.
- **Stay Hydrated:** Drinking water can help ease hunger pangs and keep you feeling full. Plus, it's good for you!
- **Review and Tweak:** Look back at your fasting schedule every few weeks. Are there consistent times when you struggle? Consider making a permanent shift.

Remember, you decide how IF integrates into your life. It's flexible. Your fasting schedule can (and should) change with your lifestyle changes! The key is to find a rhythm that feels right for you and your body.

How to Improve Your Fasting Method to Hit Various Health Goals

Intermittent fasting is versatile, and with some know-how, you can tweak it to reach your health goals better. Here are some important things to consider:

Weight Loss:

Increasing your fasting window can make a noticeable difference for those mainly looking to lose weight. A method like the 18:6, where you fast for 18 hours and only eat within a 6-hour window, could be much more effective. During these eating periods, focusing on meals that balance protein, healthy fats, and complex carbohydrates is vital. Also, maintaining a food diary can be a helpful tool, too! It allows you to track your food intake and better understand what works best for you.

Energy Boost:

Getting a boost in your energy often depends on the quality of food your body receives. When you break your fast, it's important to center your meals around nutrient-dense foods. As we've mentioned before, lean proteins like chicken or tofu paired with healthy fats like those found in avocados offer a consistent release of energy, helping you stay alert and fueled. Remember, staying hydrated is essential. Dehydration can be a sneaky cause of fatigue, so aiming for 8-10 glasses of water every day is a must!

Detox and Cleanse:

Some people decide to adopt intermittent fasting with detoxification in mind. They want to give their digestive system a well-deserved rest. During fasting, hydration becomes even more vital. It's not only about maintaining energy levels but also about helping your body flush out toxins. Drinking herbal teas, especially green or dandelion tea, can help the detoxification process. When it's time to eat, foods known for their detoxifying properties, such as garlic, beets, and lemons, should also be on the menu.

Mental Clarity:

Gaining enhanced cognitive power and a sharper mind is another benefit that many women hope to attain during their fasting journey. The best way to achieve this is by avoiding foods filled with sugar or highly processed foods. These types of food can lead to energy dips and brain fog. Instead, prioritize brain-nourishing choices like blueberries, walnuts, and nutrient-rich leafy greens. Consider incorporating practices like meditation or mindfulness into your routine to enhance your mental boost.

Overall Well-being:

Ensuring you get enough rest, dedicating time to regular physical activity, and effectively managing stress can all help elevate your health and give you the most out of your fasting program. Even simple activities like daily walks can boost your overall well-being when combined with a fasting routine.

Customization:

Remember, everyone's body and needs are unique. Ensuring your fasting approach reflects this individuality and meets your specific needs and goals is crucial. Rather than rigidly sticking to one method, feel free to adapt whenever you think it's necessary. We've said it before, but it's worth saying again: the key is to listen to your body. If something feels wrong or you're not seeing the desired results, tweak your approach accordingly.

Tailoring Fasting to Individual Lifestyles for Consistent Health Benefits

Did you know that one of the most significant benefits of intermittent fasting is that you can mold it to fit perfectly with your lifestyle? A fasting rhythm is perfect whether you're a morning person, have late-night work shifts, or enjoy evening gatherings.

First, take a moment to think about your typical day. When do you naturally feel hungrier? You may not be a breakfast person, so starting your eating window later in the day can work for you. Or perhaps you have family dinners you don't want to miss; then, consider shifting your window to include that important time.

Second, listen to your body. What is it telling you? How are you feeling? Adjust your eating window by an hour if you need a change. You're not locked into any fixed schedule. Making alterations is okay!

Remember, the goal isn't just weight loss. It's about overall health and well-being. So, consider how fasting can support your body, mental health, social life, and daily routines. With the proper adjustments and a little patience, you can make intermittent fasting a seamless and rewarding part of your life.

STRATEGIES FOR OVERCOMING PLATEAUS

No road trip is complete without a few bumps in the road. Intermittent fasting is the same! One of the most common bumps that people face is hitting a plateau. Trust me; it can feel frustrating when the scale doesn't move, or the health benefits seem to stall. But remember, plateaus are a natural part of any weight loss or health journey. They're not a sign that you're doing something wrong; instead, they indicate that it's time to reassess and tweak your actions. Recognizing a plateau and understanding how to address it can make all the difference and help you continue on your path to better health and well-being.

Identifying a Plateau

You've been diligent with your intermittent fasting routine, but lately, it feels like things have come to a standstill. So, how do you know if you've truly hit a plateau with your intermittent fasting? First, give it some time. A few days or even a week without change is not unusual, and various factors can have an influence, including water retention or fluctuations in your hormone levels. However, if weeks go by and there's still no movement on the scale, or you don't feel the usual energy levels, you've likely reached a plateau. It's also worth noting that as you lose weight, your body requires fewer calories, so overeating can slow your progress. Everyone's body reacts differently, and what might be a plateau for one person might be a natural progression for another. The key is to listen to your body, stay informed, and adjust whenever needed.

Tips for Revving Your Metabolism and Re-Igniting Weight Loss

It can be frustrating when weight loss stalls, but don't lose hope. Reigniting your metabolism and breaking through that plateau is easily achievable with a few smart techniques.

- **Adjust Your Eating Window:** If you're used to a 16-hour fast, try shifting to a 14-hour or even an 18-hour fast for a week. This slight change can kickstart your metabolism.
- **Stay Hydrated:** Water not only keeps you full but also boosts your metabolic rate. Drink plenty of water throughout the day, especially during your fasting window.
- **Up Your Protein Intake:** Ensure you consume enough protein when you break your fast. It supports muscle growth, and maintaining muscle can increase your resting metabolic rate.
- **Incorporate Strength Training:** Building muscle is a fantastic way to boost metabolism. Even simple resistance exercises using your body weight can increase your muscle mass and significantly affect your body's muscle composition.
- **Stay Active:** Beyond scheduled workouts, try to move more throughout the day. Whether it's a walk during your lunch break, stretching, or taking the stairs, any activity helps burn more calories.

- **Evaluate Your Caloric Intake:** As you lose weight, your body might need fewer calories. Ensure you're eating enough to sustain your activity levels but not so much that it hinders weight loss.
- **Practice Mindful Eating:** Pay attention to what you eat. Opt for whole foods and minimize processed items. Nutrient-dense foods can support metabolism and overall health.

What to Eat to Overcome Your Plateau

When you experience a plateau during intermittent fasting, selecting the right foods can help you break through. First, be sure to prioritize protein. Including lean meats like chicken, turkey, tofu, or fish in your meals can help repair your muscles and promote their growth.

Next, focus on fiber-rich foods. Veggies, fruits, and whole grains keep you full, support digestion, and keep your bowels moving regularly, pushing out toxins. Healthy fats from sources like avocados, nuts, and olive oil can provide long-lasting energy and keep you feeling fuller for longer. It's also essential to limit sugar and processed foods. These can cause spikes in blood sugar and might stall your weight loss progress.

Lastly, always listen to your body. Pay attention to how different foods make you feel and adjust your diet accordingly. By making these optimal dietary choices, you'll be better positioned to break through that plateau and keep progressing toward better health!

Overcoming My Personal Plateau

I remember hitting my own plateau during my fifth month of intermittent fasting. The excitement of the initial weight drop had started to wane, and I felt stuck, unable to drop even a pound for weeks. It felt like walking against a strong gust of wind – no matter how hard I pushed, I wasn't getting anywhere!

That's when doubt began to creep in. "Was intermittent fasting just another fad? Was I doing something wrong?" But then I remembered why I started this journey: my love for health and the goal to find a sustainable lifestyle change. So, I decided to experiment. I researched, adjusted my fasting hours, played around with my meals, and, most importantly, listened to my body.

What really made a difference was when I incorporated strength training into my routine and focused on nutrient-dense foods. The scales slowly began to move again. But more than the weight, I felt a surge of energy again; my skin brightened, and my moods seemed to stabilize.

That's when I realized that plateaus weren't roadblocks but opportunities to learn, adapt, and grow! This experience taught me patience, resilience, and the importance of looking beyond the scales to appreciate all the other benefits that intermittent fasting brought into my life.

Making IF a Permanent Lifestyle

For many people, intermittent fasting starts as a short-term experiment, but its potential benefits can guide you toward making it a lifelong choice. You've seen the changes, felt the energy, and perhaps even reached your weight goals. But now, it's about more than just trying it out. It's about weaving IF into the fabric of your everyday life and letting it naturally become your go-to health partner. This journey is all about evolving from a temporary phase to a sustained, enriching lifestyle.

Pros and cons: How long should you practice intermittent fasting?

You are the one in control here. You have the freedom to decide how long you want to follow this regimen. As you consider making it a significant part of your routine, let's weigh the pros and cons to see if long-term IF fits your lifestyle and health goals.

✚ Pros:

- **Sustained Weight Management:** Maintaining your desired weight becomes much easier once you find your rhythm.
- **Consistent Energy Levels:** Over time, many people experience stable energy throughout the day without the usual afternoon slumps.
- **Adaptability:** With various IF methods to choose from, you can adjust your fasting windows to better fit your daily activities and commitments.

━ Cons:

- **Initial Adjustment Phase:** Extending IF might mean undergoing another adjustment phase as your body gets used to longer fasting durations.
- **Potential Nutrient Gaps:** Relying only on limited eating windows can sometimes result in missing out on essential nutrients if not planned correctly.
- **Social Challenges:** Longer fasting windows might occasionally clash with social events or family gatherings.

Long-Term Benefits and Potential Risks of Permanent Intermittent Fasting

As you continue with intermittent fasting, it's essential to recognize the lasting benefits and be aware of potential risks. Over time, many women, like myself, have experienced the amazing transformative impact of IF, making it more than just a trend.

Benefits of Permanent IF:

- **Sustained Weight Management:** One of the top reasons many of you choose IF is for weight loss. IF can help manage and maintain a healthy weight long-term when practiced consistently.
- **Metabolic Health Boost:** IF can improve insulin sensitivity, crucial for regulating blood sugar levels. This benefit reduces the risk of type 2 diabetes.
- **Heart Health:** Regular fasting has shown positive effects on blood pressure, cholesterol levels, and other cardiovascular risk factors.
- **Brain Health:** IF boosts brain health by increasing brain-derived neurotrophic factor (BDNF), a protein linked to cognitive function and mental well-being.
- **Cellular Health:** Fasting triggers autophagy, a process where cells remove damaged components, promoting cellular repair and function.

Potential Risks:

- **Nutrient Deficiency:** Extended fasting without careful planning can lead to inadequate nutrient intake. It's vital to eat balanced meals during your eating windows.

- **Overeating:** Some might feel extremely hungry after a fasting period, leading to overconsumption during eating windows.
- **Mental Well-being:** IF might not suit everyone. For some, it can lead to increased stress, obsession with food, or even eating disorders.
- **Potential Health Complications:** While IF can offer numerous benefits, consulting with a healthcare professional is essential, especially if you have underlying health conditions.

EMBRACING A LIFELONG COMMITMENT TO INTERMITTENT FASTING

Transitioning to an intermittent fasting lifestyle might feel challenging at first. Over time, this lifestyle integrates easily into your daily routine. Especially for women over 50, adopting IF long-term offers numerous health benefits and can become a habit for forming the foundation of a healthy lifestyle.

- **Consistency is your best friend.** Like any good habit, the more regularly you practice IF, the more natural it becomes. You might naturally skip breakfast or not feel the need to snack late at night. It's about understanding and listening to your body's hunger cues.
- **It's also essential to stay informed.** New research about IF surfaces regularly. Keeping yourself updated helps you make informed choices and switch up your IF approach for the best possible outcomes. Joining an IF community, whether online or offline, can offer support, allow you to share updates, and provide a platform for discussing concerns or sharing your success.

- **Flexibility is key.** There will be days when you'll want to adjust your fasting window because of travel, special events, or changes in your schedule. It's okay! IF isn't about rigid rules; it's about finding a system that works for you, accommodating life's unpredictable nature.
- **Lastly, cherish the journey.** Every step you take towards maintaining your IF lifestyle is a step towards better health and well-being. Celebrate the small wins, learn from the setbacks, and always remember why you started this journey in the first place. Your commitment to IF is a testament to your dedication to a healthier, happier you.

My Personal Journey to an Enduring IF Lifestyle

I'll be honest; I was skeptical when I first heard about intermittent fasting. The idea of not eating for extended periods sounded scary, especially when, like many, I was used to the traditional three meals a day (with my fair share of snacks in between!). However, as I began to look into it, I realized that there were a lot of benefits for women like myself, so being the adventurous type, I decided to give it a try!

The first few weeks were challenging. I missed my morning toast and my late-night snacking. But as the days went by, I started noticing some changes. My weight was dropping, I had a ton of energy, and my digestive issues (which were an issue for years) were starting to subside. I couldn't believe it!

But the real test came when life threw me a bunch of curveballs like my niece's unexpected evening wedding, the spontaneous brunch invites, or that weekend getaway where the hotel's breakfast spread was too good to skip. Initially, I thought these interruptions meant failure. But instead of giving up, I adapted.

I learned that flexibility was key. So, I began adjusting my fasting hours. Some days, I'd start early, while others, I'd push my eating window further into the evening.

Accepting intermittent fasting as a part of my lifestyle also meant continuously learning about it. I joined IF groups, attended webinars, and read up on the latest research. These connections not only kept me updated but reinforced my commitment.

Today, years into my IF journey, I can confidently say that it's become an integral part of my life. Yes, there are days when I falter and some when I don't practice IF at all, but these are few and far between. Most days, I feel on top of the world! It's all a part of the journey. With patience, flexibility, and understanding, adopting IF as a lifelong commitment can be a rewarding experience.

Taking the Next Steps of Your IF Journey

Intermittent fasting doesn't just have to be a temporary phase of your life; it can evolve into a fulfilling, lifelong journey. This chapter explored the foundations of integrating IF into your daily routines, ensuring consistency, and tailoring it to suit your unique needs. From understanding plateaus to the advantages of daily time-restricted fasting methods, you now have the tools to make intermittent fasting a seamless part of your health routine. One of the most important things we looked at is its potential for longevity and adaptability, especially how this relates to the unique challenges faced by women over 50.

Our journey through the world of intermittent fasting will get even more fascinating. In the upcoming pages, we will look at menopause, emotional well-being, and how all of this comes into play with intermittent fasting. As women over 50, some unique challenges and changes come with menopause. But, with the proper knowledge and strategies, you can confidently navigate this phase of your life, using intermittent fasting as a powerful ally.

9

S: SPECIAL CONSIDERATIONS FOR WOMEN OVER 50

When you first started intermittent fasting, it may have felt like a phase that you wanted to kickstart your health. But as you've moved forward, I've shown you all of its tremendous potential. IF isn't just some fad that will disappear faster than a slice of pumpkin pie at Thanksgiving. It's here to stay and can be a part of your daily routine for years to come. As we navigate the significant "change" that every woman must go through, IF can be your trusted BFF. You already know how it can help you lose weight and boost your health. Now, we will look at how intermittent fasting can help you navigate the new terrain of menopause.

MENOPAUSE AND IF

Menopause is a natural stage in every woman's life character-ized by significant hormonal changes. As your body adjusts to these changes, you might notice changes in your metabolism, energy levels, and weight. Intermittent fasting can be a helpful ally during this time. Let's look at how we can tailor IF to work best for you during and after menopause.

Implementing IF During the Different Stages of Menopause

When I started my intermittent fasting journey, I was already familiar with the challenges of menopause. As women, we have to endure many different stages of menopause, and each one comes with a unique set of challenges. Understanding these stages and customizing your IF approach can make a world of difference to how you feel during this time.

- **Perimenopause:** This is the transition phase leading up to menopause, often starting in your late 40s. Hormone levels slowly begin to fluctuate, which can cause irregular periods, mood swings, and even unexpected weight gain. During this time, starting with a more flexible IF schedule, like the 12:12 method, can be beneficial. It can help ease your body into a fasting routine without adding extra stress to an already stressful time.
- **Menopause:** Generally occurring in the early 50s, this is when your periods stop altogether. With the decline of estrogen, many women experience hot flashes, mood changes, and difficulty sleeping. It's also a time when unwanted weight can start to accumulate around your midsection. I personally adjusted my IF schedule during this period, opting for a 14:10 window. Adapting gave my body adequate fasting time while still being gentle.
- **Postmenopause:** This stage comes about a year after the last period. The symptoms of menopause may lessen, but the risk of health conditions like osteoporosis increases due to the lower estrogen levels. At this point, many women feel comfortable enough to try a 16:8 IF schedule. Pack your meals with calcium-rich foods to support your bone health during this time.

Regardless of the stage of menopause you are in, it's essential to listen to your body. Adjust your fasting windows based on how you feel. Remember to consult a healthcare professional, especially if you're new to IF. And as always, prioritize nutrient-rich foods that support hormonal balance and overall health. It might be a bit challenging at first, but with patience and consistency, you can make IF work for you throughout your menopausal journey.

SPECIAL NUTRITIONAL NEEDS

As we cross the 50-year mark, our body's nutritional needs start to shift. I've learned firsthand that our metabolism slows, and the risk for certain health issues increases. But with proper nutrition, you can support your body's changing needs and feel vibrant and healthy no matter what changes your body is going through.

In my own journey, I placed a special emphasis on calcium and vitamin D for bone health. Omega-3 fatty acids from sources like fish and flaxseed help heart health. Fiber-rich foods like whole grains, fruits, and veggies support digestion and help manage weight. Additionally, lean proteins from chicken, fish, beans, or tofu are crucial to help maintain muscle mass.

With age, you may also notice a reduced appetite. However, it's essential not to skip meals. Instead, opt for smaller, nutrient-rich meals and snacks throughout the day. Limiting processed foods and increasing my water intake has also benefited me. The results include diminished bloating and a notable enhancement in my digestive health.

Tips and Dietary Advice:

- Maintaining a balanced diet and considering foods that stabilize blood sugar is crucial for preventing diabetes.
- Including protein in every meal will help counter muscle loss.
- Be mindful of calorie intake. I found that needing fewer calories was a reality after 50, so being aware can prevent unwanted weight gain through unnecessary overeating.
- Dairy products or calcium-fortified foods daily helped maintain my bone strength.
- Reading labels is essential so that you know exactly what you are eating.
- Finally, variety is key. I made it a point to add colorful fruits and veggies to my plate, ensuring I get a range of nutrients to support overall health.

FINDING EMOTIONAL WELL-BEING AND SUPPORT SYSTEMS

Trying to tackle the ups and downs of menopause while practicing intermittent fasting can be an emotional roller coaster. I've felt that and know precisely how challenging it can be! Hormonal fluctuations can affect mood, energy, and stress levels, making prioritizing emotional well-being paramount during this time.

Having a positive mindset has been my anchor. Starting each day with gratitude, focusing on my achievements rather than setbacks, and practicing meditation have all been game-changers. Whenever I started to feel stress creeping in, I turned my attention to activities I love – like a brisk walk or journaling my feelings. Doing these things helped to center myself and took my attention away from my stress.

Surrounding yourself with supportive friends and family is also invaluable. During my low days, I found comfort in sharing my experiences, frustrations, and successes with close friends. Having someone who listens and understands what you are going through can make all the difference. There were days when intermittent fasting felt challenging, especially when I was also experiencing those intense menopause symptoms. On one of these days, I felt so overwhelmed. Instead of internalizing my feelings, I called up a close friend. We talked and laughed; by the end, I felt lighter and more motivated. It was a clear reminder of how vital emotional well-being is and how a robust support system can uplift us.

Tips for Prioritizing Mental Health:

- Remember, it's okay to seek professional guidance. I've benefited from counseling sessions, especially when menopause felt overwhelming.
- Celebrate small victories. Whether it's sticking to your IF schedule or walking that extra mile, every achievement counts.
- Stay connected. Regularly check in with loved ones, and don't hesitate to express your feelings.
- Attend support groups or online forums. Interacting with like-minded people on a similar journey can be insightful and comforting.
- Take time out for yourself. Setting aside some "me time" can help you reset and give you the break you need to push forward through any challenges.

From Knowledge to Nourishment - Taking the Next Steps

As we wrap up this chapter, let's take just a moment to reflect on our journey together this far. We've explored the relationship between menopause, nutrition, and intermittent fasting. Embracing the changes menopause brings while ensuring we nourish our bodies and minds is essential. Remember, intermittent fasting isn't just a phase—it's a lifestyle choice that can significantly support you during this unique time of your life. Trust me, I've been there. I have faced the same challenges and witnessed firsthand the fantastic ways that IF can make a difference during the change. You've got this!

As we shift our focus to the next chapter, we will venture into the world of delicious recipes tailored to your specific needs. Get ready to start your 29-day meal plan that not only aligns with your intermittent fasting goals but also tantalizes your taste buds. Good food and good health await!

10

E: ENLIGHTENMENT WITH YOUR 29-DAY MEAL PLAN

Navigating the world of nutrition, especially when adding intermittent fasting to the mix, can feel like solving a complicated and confusing puzzle. But guess what? You've already laid down most of the pieces. Now, it's about fitting them together to see the beautiful (and healthy!) picture they create. Nutrition is not just about keeping hunger at bay; it's the cornerstone of our health.

You've spent time learning about intermittent fasting and its endless benefits. Let's focus on the equally important part: what you eat during your eating windows. It's like fueling a car: the quality of the fuel impacts performance. Your body, during fasting, gears up to absorb and use nutrients efficiently once you decide to break your fast. And just like you wouldn't put any random fuel into a luxury car, you shouldn't put just any food into your body. The recipes I've shared are designed to give you high-quality fuel: nutritious, balanced, and, most importantly, delicious meals!

Over the years, I've realized that sticking to a healthy eating routine doesn't feel like a chore when our meals are colorful, tasty, and packed with nutrition. Instead, it becomes a delicious and delightful experience. We have formulated every recipe here to include a balanced amount of protein, healthy fats, and necessary vitamins and minerals.

But here's the fun part - it's totally flexible! Everyone's tastes and needs are unique. So, feel free to mix and match these recipes. Create a meal plan that resonates with you, ensuring every day is a culinary delight and a step towards your health goals. Remember, this journey is all about celebrating you, and what better way than with food that loves you back?

29 BREAKFAST RECIPES

Smoothies

1. **Berry Bliss Smoothie:** Start with a cup of mixed berries: blueberries, strawberries, and raspberries. Add half a banana for a smooth texture. Add almond milk for a creamy base, and sprinkle a tablespoon of chia seeds for fiber. Blend until smooth. You get a vibrant, berry-packed drink that's a delightful morning kickstart.

2. **Tropical Sunrise:** Use generous chunks of mango and pineapple. Blend with coconut milk for a rich tropical taste. Add a small spoonful of honey for sweetness. This smoothie tastes like a tropical island escape, ensuring a bright start to your day.

3. **Green Goddess Smoothie:** Mix a handful of spinach with half an avocado and a cored apple. Use water as your base. This results in a refreshing, light green drink perfect for those seeking a healthy boost without any heaviness.

4. **Creamy Peanut Butter Delight:** Take a ripe banana and two tablespoons of peanut butter and blend with almond milk. Add a touch of cocoa powder for that chocolatey twist. It's a blend that feels like a dessert but is perfect for breakfast.

5. **Golden Glow Turmeric Smoothie:** Add a teaspoon of turmeric and ginger to half a banana and coconut milk. This smoothie has a vibrant golden hue, making it a treat for the eyes and a health booster for your body.

6. **Choco-Mint Cooler:** Choose a ripe banana blend with two tablespoons of cocoa powder, almond milk, and a few drops of mint extract. It's a refreshing and satisfying smoothie, especially for chocolate lovers.

7. **Sweet Cinnamon Oat Delight:** Start with half a cup of oats. Add almond milk, a pinch of cinnamon, and a drizzle of honey. Blend until creamy. It's a drink that fills you up and keeps you energized for hours.

8. **Zesty Orange Creamsicle:** Blend fresh orange slices with a cup of Greek yogurt. Add a drop of vanilla extract and honey to enhance the taste. It's a citrusy, creamy delight that awakens the senses.

9. **Velvety Vanilla Almond:** Combine almond milk, two table-spoons of almond butter, a banana, and a drop of vanilla extract. What you get is an ultra-smooth, nutty, and rich drink that's bound to become a favorite.

10. **Cool Cucumber Refresher:** Use half a cucumber, sliced. Add it to Greek yogurt, a splash of lime juice, and a hint of honey. Blend and enjoy. It's crisp, fresh, and just what you need on a warm day or post-workout.

Smoothie Bowls

11. **Berry Burst Bowl:** Kickstart with a blend of blueberries, raspberries, and strawberries, using almond milk for a thick, creamy base. Once it achieves a spoonable consistency, pour it into a bowl. For that added crunch, top with granola, chia seeds, and coconut flakes. Dive in for a berry-intense experience, a beautiful fusion of flavors and textures, ensuring you get both delight and nutrients in each bite.

12 **Tropical Oasis Bowl:** Bring the tropics to your breakfast table. Start with a mix of juicy mango chunks and fresh pineapple slices, blending them with coconut milk for a rich taste. Pour into a bowl and garnish with kiwi slices, toasted coconut, and a drizzle of honey. It's like a vacation in a bowl - bright, sunny, and refreshing.

13. **Chocolate Dream Bowl:** For those indulgent mornings, blend a ripe banana with cocoa powder and almond milk until smooth and creamy. Pour your chocolatey blend into a bowl and finish with toppings like dark chocolate chips, almond slices, and a sprinkle of oats. It's a decadent treat that will satiate your sweet cravings while being a healthy choice.

14. **Green Vitality Bowl:** Using fresh spinach, kale, and half an avocado, blend these greens with a splash of apple juice until thick and creamy. Transfer to a bowl and get creative with toppings like pumpkin seeds, goji berries, and a swirl of yogurt. It's a bowl full of vitality, ensuring you start the day with a dose of health and flavor.

15. **Peanut Butter Power Bowl:** This is for protein seekers. Blend together a scoop of your favorite protein powder, banana, and generous dollops of peanut butter with oat milk. Once creamy, pour into a bowl and garnish with banana slices, a sprinkle of granola, and a drizzle of more peanut butter.

Energizing and satisfying, it's the fuel you need for a busy day ahead.

Oatmeal

16. **Cinnamon Apple Delight:** Begin by simmering rolled oats in almond milk. Mix in finely diced apples and a sprinkle of cinnamon as they soften. Continue to cook until you reach a creamy consistency. Once done, serve in a bowl and top with toasted walnuts, a drizzle of honey, and an extra dash of cinnamon. This bowl promises a heartwarming flavor, reminiscent of apple pie, but with the added benefit of being wholesome.

17. **Tropical Coconut Bliss:** Prepare your oats using a mixture of water and coconut milk for a creamier texture. When halfway done, fold in diced pineapple and shredded coconut. Once ready, pour into a bowl and garnish with a few mango slices, more shredded coconut, and a splash of coconut milk. Each spoonful transports you to a tropical paradise while nourishing your body.

18. **Berry Medley Morning:** Slow-cook your oats in oat milk, adding a touch of vanilla extract. As they're almost ready, fold in a mix of raspberries, blueberries, and blackberries. Serve in your favorite bowl, finishing with a dollop of Greek yogurt, a sprinkle of chia seeds, and a few more fresh berries on top. It's a berry-packed start to the day, balancing sweetness, tartness, and nutrition.

19. **Chocolate and Banana Dream:** Infuse your morning oats with a spoon of cocoa powder while cooking them in cashew milk. Once creamy, stir in slices of ripe banana and a touch of maple syrup. Serve in a bowl with a garnish of dark chocolate shavings, a few banana slices, and a sprinkle of flaxseeds. This

bowl combines indulgence with health, making mornings feel like a treat.

20. **Savory Spinach and Mushroom Oats:** For a savory twist, sauté chopped garlic, sliced mushrooms, and baby spinach in a pan. Set aside and cook your oats in vegetable broth until creamy. Mix the sautéed veggies into the oats, seasoning with a pinch of salt and pepper. Serve hot, garnished with a sprinkle of grated parmesan and a few cherry tomatoes. It's a comforting and hearty bowl, perfect for those who lean towards savory breakfasts.

Breakfast Muffins and Loaves

21. **Zesty Lemon Blueberry Muffins:** Whip whole wheat flour, baking powder, a hint of salt, and a dash of cinnamon. Gently fold in fresh blueberries. In another bowl, mix Greek yogurt, honey, egg, vanilla extract, and lemon zest. Combine both mixtures until just blended. Pour into muffin tins and bake until golden. The result? Moist, tangy muffins with bursts of blueberries. Perfect with your morning coffee or tea.

22. **Chia Seed and Banana Loaf:** Blend ripe bananas, honey, vanilla extract, and two eggs until smooth. Gradually incorporate whole wheat flour, baking soda, a pinch of salt, and a handful of chia seeds. Pour the batter into a loaf pan and sprinkle with more chia seeds. Bake to perfection. Every slice offers the subtle sweetness of bananas combined with the crunch of chia, making for a filling, nutritious start.

23. **Carrot and Walnut Muffins:** Begin with grated carrots, crushed walnuts, and raisins in a bowl. In another, whisk whole wheat flour, baking powder, cinnamon, and nutmeg. Combine both with Greek yogurt, honey, and two beaten eggs. Pour into muffin molds and bake until they're a beautiful golden brown.

These muffins bring a delightful crunch and are packed with the natural sweetness of carrots and raisins.

24. **Pumpkin Spice Loaf:** Embrace autumn vibes by mixing pumpkin puree, maple syrup, vanilla extract, and eggs in a bowl. Gradually blend in whole wheat flour, baking soda, and a blend of cinnamon, nutmeg, and ginger. Transfer the batter to a loaf pan and bake. This loaf is a cozy, spiced delight, with each slice offering the rich, comforting taste of pumpkin. Perfect for crisp mornings.

Egg White Recipes

While these recipes call for just the egg whites, feel free to include the yolk occasionally as desired. It is filled with extra calories and fats and can help keep you feeling fuller for longer.

25. **Mediterranean Egg White Omelette:** Start by sautéing diced tomatoes, spinach, olives, and crumbled feta in a non-stick pan. Pour in whisked egg whites seasoned with a pinch of salt and pepper. Let it set, fold, and serve. This omelet transports you straight to the Mediterranean shores with its vibrant flavors and healthy ingredients.

26. **Egg White and Avocado Wraps:** In a skillet, cook seasoned egg whites until set, stirring occasionally. Lay out a whole-grain tortilla, spread some mashed avocado, sprinkle a touch of chili flakes, and place the cooked egg whites in the center. Roll up and enjoy. This wrap is a creamy, spicy blend of healthy fats and proteins — a refreshing way to start your day.

27. **Spinach and Mushroom Egg White Frittata:** Sauté sliced mushrooms and fresh spinach in olive oil. Season and add in beaten egg whites. Transfer to the oven and bake until set. This frittata is a low-carb, high-protein dish packed with earthy flavors and nutritious greens.

28. **Egg White Breakfast Cups:** In muffin tins, layer diced bell peppers, spinach, and a touch of grated cheddar. Pour seasoned egg whites into each cup and bake until firm. These breakfast cups are colorful, portable, and filled with a delightful mix of textures and tastes.

29. **Egg White and Quinoa Scramble:** Cook quinoa and set aside. In a pan, scramble egg whites with a dash of salt and pepper. Once almost set, mix in the quinoa and sprinkle some chopped parsley. This high-protein scramble is a delicious fusion of fluffy egg whites and nutty quinoa, ensuring a filling and balanced start to your day.

LUNCH RECIPES

Salads

1. **Classic Caesar with Grilled Chicken:** Crisp romaine lettuce, grilled chicken strips, homemade whole-grain croutons, and shaved parmesan cheese. Drizzle with a tangy Caesar dressing made from Greek yogurt, lemon juice, garlic, and anchovy paste. This salad is a hearty classic with a burst of flavors.

2. **Mediterranean Tuna Salad:** Mix flaked canned tuna, sliced cucumber, cherry tomatoes, olives, red onion, and crumbled feta. Serve with a dressing of olive oil, red wine vinegar, oregano, and lemon zest. Dive into the refreshing flavors of the Mediterranean with every bite.

3. **Steak and Arugula Salad:** Thinly sliced, medium-rare grilled steak atop peppery arugula, roasted cherry tomatoes, and crumbled blue cheese finished with a balsamic reduction glaze. This recipe is a luxurious salad that satisfies every meat lover's dream.

4. **Asian-inspired Shrimp Salad:** Sautéed shrimp, shredded carrots, sliced bell peppers, edamame, and crispy wonton strips on a bed of mixed greens. A dressing of sesame oil, lime juice, soy sauce, and honey ties it all together—an East Asian delicacy on a plate.

5. **Chickpea and Feta Delight:** Hearty chickpeas, diced bell peppers, red onion, cherry tomatoes, and crumbled feta cheese. Combine with a simple olive oil, lemon juice, and fresh mint dressing. This salad is a delightful mix of textures and Mediterranean flavors.

6. **Quinoa and Black Bean Fiesta:** Cooked quinoa, black beans, sweet corn, diced avocado, cherry tomatoes, and a sprinkle of cilantro. Drizzle with a zesty lime and cumin dressing. A protein-packed salad with vibrant Southwestern flavors.

7. **Grilled Salmon Spinach Salad:** Flaky grilled salmon atop fresh baby spinach with red onion, avocado slices, and toasted almond slivers. Serve with a dill, lemon juice, and olive oil dressing. It's a culinary delight that doesn't compromise on health benefits.

8. **Turkey and Cranberry Green Salad:** Sliced roasted turkey breast, dried cranberries, goat cheese crumbles, and walnut pieces on mixed greens. Toss with a maple-mustard vinaigrette for a festive touch. A salad that brings holiday flavors all year round.

9. **Lentil and Goat Cheese Salad:** Tender green lentils, beetroot wedges, baby spinach, and creamy goat cheese rounds. Dress with a tangy apple cider vinegar, olive oil, and thyme concoction. It's a rustic and hearty lunch option.

10. **Thai Beef Salad:** Slices of grilled beef steak, mixed greens, julienned carrots, cucumber, and fresh mint leaves. Drench with a dressing made of fish sauce, lime juice, brown sugar, and a

touch of chili. This tantalizing salad dances between sweet, sour, and savory.

Sandwiches and Wraps

11. Roasted Veggie and Hummus Wrap: Spread creamy hummus on a whole-grain wrap. Top with roasted bell peppers, zucchini, eggplant slices, and baby spinach. Roll tightly and slice in half. It's a mouthwatering wrap that packs a flavorful punch of roasted goodness with every bite.

12. Turkey, Apple, and Brie Sandwich: Layer thin slices of smoked turkey, crisp apple slices, and creamy brie cheese between multigrain bread. Grill until the cheese is slightly melted and the bread is golden. The sandwich strikes a delightful balance of smoky, sweet, and creamy.

13. Spicy Chicken Caesar Wrap: Fill a spinach tortilla with grilled chicken strips tossed in spicy buffalo sauce. Add crisp romaine lettuce, shaved parmesan, and a drizzle of Caesar dressing. Roll up for a zesty twist on the classic Caesar in a portable wrap form.

14. Mediterranean Veggie and Feta Sandwich: Spread a layer of olive tapenade on toasted ciabatta bread. Stack with sliced cucumbers, red onion rings, juicy tomatoes, and crumbled feta cheese. Top with a drizzle of olive oil and a sprinkle of oregano. This sandwich is a sunny Mediterranean day in each bite.

15. Tuna Salad Croissant Wrap: Mix flaked tuna with diced celery, a dollop of Greek yogurt, fresh dill, lemon zest, and a pinch of black pepper. Spread the mix generously over a soft croissant. Add lettuce and thinly sliced cucumber for crunch. It is a sophisticated and creamy delight, perfect for a classy lunch.

Flatbreads

16. Mediterranean Pita: Spread roasted red pepper hummus on the top of a pita. Top with grilled chicken pieces, juicy cherry tomatoes, crumbled feta cheese, and a sprinkle of fresh parsley. Pair this with a side of tangy tzatziki sauce and crisp cucumber sticks. A bite of this pita whisks you straight to the Mediterranean coast.

17. Spiced Lamb on Naan: Layer tender, spiced lamb slices over a piece of soft naan bread. Drizzle with mint-yogurt sauce and garnish with pickled red onions and fresh cilantro leaves. For a side, enjoy a cooling carrot and raisin salad, giving a sweet crunch to contrast the spiced lamb.

18. BBQ Chicken Tortilla Crunch: Spread a thin layer of smoky BBQ sauce on a whole wheat tortilla. Top with shredded BBQ chicken, thinly sliced red onions, and a sprinkle of cheddar cheese. Warm until cheese is melty. Cut into wedges and serve with a refreshing corn and black bean salad, adding a zesty zest to the smoky main.

19. Asian-inspired Shrimp Flatbread: Place marinated, grilled shrimp on a toasted sesame flatbread. Drizzle with a sweet chili-mayo sauce, then garnish with sliced scallions and fresh cilantro. As a side, a crunchy Asian slaw with red cabbage, julienned carrots, and a sprinkle of sesame seeds complements the shrimp's sweetness.

20. Mushroom and Goat Cheese Focaccia: Spread a layer of creamy goat cheese on a slice of focaccia bread—top with sautéed mushrooms, caramelized onions, and fresh rosemary. Drizzle with truffle oil for a rich finish. This lunch, complemented by vinaigrette-mixed greens, strikes a balance between earthy and sophisticated.

Soups and Stews

21. Classic Chicken Noodle Soup: Dive into a bowl of comforting chicken noodle soup, where tender chunks of chicken meet curly egg noodles in a savory broth infused with bay leaves, thyme, and a hint of garlic. The flavors mingle together, creating that timeless taste of home. Serve it alongside oven-toasted garlic bread, crispy on the outside and soft on the inside, making every bite a cozy embrace.

22. Creamy Tomato Basil Soup: Immerse yourself in the rich, velvety texture of this tomato basil soup. Sun-ripened tomatoes blend seamlessly with a touch of cream and fragrant basil, giving you a sip of Mediterranean summer. For the side, enjoy a crunchy Caesar salad with crisp romaine, shaved parmesan, and a sprinkle of croutons, adding a contrasting bite to the creamy soup.

23. Hearty Beef and Vegetable Stew: Relish a robust beef stew where chunks of slow-cooked beef meld with carrots, potatoes, and green beans in a flavorful, herb-infused broth. This stew is the epitome of hearty satisfaction. Pair this with a slice of freshly baked whole grain bread, perfect for soaking up that savory goodness.

24. Spicy Lentil and Spinach Soup: Dive into this vibrant, spicy lentil soup, where green lentils simmer with tomatoes, spinach, and a hint of curry. It's a bowl that promises both warmth and a delightful kick. On the side, a cool yogurt cucumber dip with a sprinkle of dill is not only refreshing but acts as the perfect cool-down companion to the spicy soup.

Lunch Bowls

25. Quinoa Fiesta Bowl: Start with a fluffy bed of protein-packed quinoa, then top it with grilled chicken strips, zesty black beans, corn, and diced red bell peppers. Drizzle with a cilantro-lime dressing, and finish with a dollop of creamy avocado. It's a burst of flavors and textures, sure to liven up your lunchtime.

26. Mediterranean Farro Delight: Dive into a bowl of nutty farro grains mixed with juicy cherry tomatoes, cucumber slices, tangy feta cheese, and Kalamata olives. A lemon-oregano dressing ties everything together, evoking those breezy Mediterranean shores. Each bite is a refreshing journey to the coast.

27. Teriyaki Chicken Brown Rice Bowl: Layer a base of earthy brown rice, then pile on tender slices of teriyaki-glazed chicken. Add steamed broccoli florets and shredded carrot for a splash of color. Top off with sesame seeds and a drizzle of extra teriyaki sauce. It's a savory and satisfying blend of East meets West.

28. Barley Veggie Bliss Bowl: Experience the chewy goodness of barley grains coupled with roasted butternut squash, charred Brussels sprouts, and sautéed mushrooms. A rosemary-infused olive oil drizzle completes this hearty veggie ensemble. This bowl sings the praises of nature's bounty in every bite.

29. Spiced Chickpea Couscous Bowl: Indulge in the light fluffiness of couscous paired with spiced roasted chickpeas, diced red onion, and bell peppers. A cumin and lemon dressing brings warmth and zing, while a sprinkle of fresh mint refreshes the palate. A delightful dance of North African flavors awaits.

DINNER RECIPES

Pasta Dishes

1. **Whole Wheat Spaghetti with Lemon-Garlic Shrimp:** Start with whole wheat spaghetti for a nutritious twist. Cook it al dente and toss it in a light sauce made of sautéed garlic, red chili flakes, and fresh shrimp. Finish with a generous squeeze of lemon juice, zest, and a handful of chopped fresh parsley. Enjoy this refreshing, zesty dish that brings the taste of the sea right to your plate.

2. **Spinach and Ricotta Stuffed Shells:** Opt for jumbo pasta shells and stuff them with a wholesome mixture of ricotta cheese, steamed spinach, and a dash of nutmeg. Lay them in a baking dish over a bed of your favorite marinara sauce, sprinkle with mozzarella, and bake until bubbly. Pair with a simple green salad for a comforting and balanced meal.

3. **Grilled Vegetable Penne with Basil Pesto:** Char-grill zucchini, bell peppers, and cherry tomatoes for a smoky flavor. Mix them with cooked penne pasta and homemade basil pesto (basil, pine nuts, garlic, olive oil, and parmesan). The combination is a delightful medley of fresh tastes and hearty satisfaction.

4. **Chicken Fettuccine in Creamy Mushroom Sauce:** Use whole grain fettuccine and toss it in a creamy sauce made from sautéed mushrooms, lean grilled chicken strips, a splash of white wine, and a touch of light cream. Garnish with fresh thyme and enjoy this rich, earthy dish that's both hearty and nourishing.

5. **Tomato and Olive Rotini with Feta:** Cook rotini pasta and mix it with a vibrant sauce of diced tomatoes, Kalamata olives, capers, and garlic, cooked down to perfection. Finish with

crumbled feta cheese and a sprinkle of fresh oregano. This Mediterranean-inspired dish is a festival of flavors, sure to please your palate.

Casseroles

6. **Quinoa and Vegetable Bake:** Begin with cooked quinoa as your hearty base, blending it with a colorful mix of sautéed bell peppers, zucchini, and cherry tomatoes. Stir in chickpeas for added protein and sprinkle with a light layer of mozzarella. Bake until golden, and you have a protein-packed, veggie-rich dish ready to serve.

7. **Chicken and Broccoli Alfredo Casserole:** Layer lean grilled chicken strips and steamed broccoli florets in a baking dish. Pour over a light Alfredo sauce made from garlic, a splash of chicken broth, Greek yogurt, and Parmesan cheese. Top with whole wheat breadcrumbs and bake until bubbly. It's creamy comfort food with a nutritious twist.

8. **Sweet Potato and Black Bean Enchilada Bake:** Layer thin slices of roasted sweet potatoes with a hearty mix of black beans, corn, and enchilada sauce. Sprinkle with a hint of cumin and chili powder, then top with Monterey Jack cheese. Once baked to perfection, garnish with fresh cilantro. This dish brings a sweet and savory fusion that's both filling and flavorful.

9. **Mediterranean Tuna Noodle Casserole:** Opt for whole wheat penne and toss it with flaked tuna, sautéed spinach, cherry tomatoes, and Kalamata olives. Add a light lemon-oregano béchamel sauce and mix well. Top with feta cheese crumbles and bake until heated through. Dive into this fresh and zesty twist on a classic.

10. **Turkey and Mushroom Rice Bake:** Mix cooked brown rice with ground turkey sautéed with onions, garlic, and sliced

mushrooms. Stir in a splash of low-sodium soy sauce and a sprinkle of fresh thyme. Place the mixture into a baking dish and cover with a layer of grated Swiss cheese. Bake until the top is melted and slightly crispy. This dish offers a delicious combination of earthy flavors and satisfying textures.

Slow Cooker Recipes

11. **Hearty Lentil and Vegetable Stew:** Begin with green lentils, rinsed and drained. Add chunks of carrots, celery, potatoes, and diced tomatoes into your slow cooker. Season with bay leaves, cumin, and a dash of smoked paprika. Pour in vegetable broth and let it simmer on low. By evening, you'll be greeted with a thick, hearty stew, bursting with earthy flavors.

12. **Tender Teriyaki Chicken:** Place chicken breasts into the slow cooker, pouring over a mix of low-sodium soy sauce, honey, minced garlic, and grated ginger. Add a touch of rice vinegar for zing. Let the flavors meld together on low. Serve the tender chicken over brown rice with a sprinkling of sesame seeds and sliced green onions.

13. **Vegetable and Chickpea Curry:** Pour coconut milk into your slow cooker, then stir in chickpeas, diced sweet potatoes, spinach, and peas. Add a blend of curry powder, turmeric, and ground coriander. Let the medley cook slowly, infusing the creamy coconut base with spicy aromas. Garnish with fresh cilantro and enjoy with a side of quinoa.

14. **Zesty Italian Beef Roast:** Nestle a lean beef roast into your slow cooker. Pour over a mix of diced tomatoes, Italian seasoning, minced garlic, and a splash of red wine. Let it cook until the meat is fork-tender. Shred and serve on whole grain rolls or with a side of steamed veggies for a rustic, Italian-inspired feast.

15. **Butternut Squash and White Bean Chili:** Combine chunks of butternut squash, white beans, corn, and diced bell peppers. Stir in a mix of vegetable broth, chili powder, and cumin. As the chili simmers, the squash turns velvety, and the beans tender. Top with a dollop of Greek yogurt and a sprinkle of cheddar for a comforting, veggie-forward bowl of goodness.

Seafood Dinners

16. **Mediterranean Salmon Bowl:** Place a salmon fillet on a baking tray seasoned with lemon zest, dill, and a touch of olive oil. Once baked to perfection, lay it atop a bed of quinoa mixed with cherry tomatoes, cucumber slices, and kalamata olives. Drizzle with a lemon-tahini dressing and garnish with feta. It's a refreshing bowl, bursting with the flavors of the Mediterranean.

17. **Zesty Shrimp Tacos:** Sauté shrimp with a hint of chili powder and cumin until pink and succulent. Spoon them onto whole grain tortillas, adding a diced mango salsa, red onion, and chopped cilantro. Finish with a squeeze of lime for that zesty punch. Serve with a side of grilled corn, making it a playful, flavor-packed dinner.

18. **Lemon Herb Tilapia:** Steam tilapia fillets with slivers of garlic, a sprinkle of dried herbs, and fresh lemon slices. Once tender and flaky, serve alongside roasted asparagus spears drizzled with a dash of olive oil. This meal is simplicity at its best, letting the clean flavors shine.

19. **Spicy Mussels in Tomato Broth:** In a pot, simmer mussels with diced tomatoes, a splash of white wine, crushed red pepper flakes, and chopped parsley. Once the mussels have opened, ladle them out with the aromatic broth. Serve with a slice of whole grain bread to soak up the spicy, tangy juices. It's a coastal treat with a kick!

20. **Seared Scallops with Spinach Pesto Pasta:** Pan-sear scallops until they have a golden crust. Toss whole-grain spaghetti with a vibrant spinach, basil, and walnut pesto. Plate the pasta and top with the seared scallops. Garnish with parmesan shavings for an elegant touch. It's a gourmet meal that's both indulgent and nourishing.

BBQ Dinners

21. **Grilled Veggie Platter:** Skewer bell peppers, zucchini, cherry tomatoes, and red onion drizzled with olive oil and seasoned with rosemary and thyme. Grill them until they're charred and tender. Serve with a tangy yogurt dip. It's a rainbow of flavors and nutrients in every bite, celebrating the garden's freshest.

22. **Honey-Lime Chicken Skewers:** Marinate chunks of chicken breast in a blend of honey, lime zest, garlic, and a dash of soy sauce. Thread them onto skewers and grill until beautifully golden. Paired with a quinoa salad, this dish brings a touch of sweet and tangy to your BBQ fare.

23. **Spicy Grilled Tofu Steaks:** Coat thick tofu slices in a spicy mix of paprika, cayenne, and a touch of maple syrup. Grill until they've got a nice crispy exterior, and serve with fresh mango and avocado salsa. This dish is a delightful fusion of heat and sweetness.

24. **BBQ Portobello Mushrooms:** Brush Portobello mushroom caps with a mixture of balsamic vinegar, minced garlic, and a sprinkle of salt and pepper. Grill them gill-side down first, turning once, until tender. Paired with a mixed greens salad, it's a meaty yet meat-free delight for the palate.

25. **Grilled Seafood Salad:** Grill shrimp and scallops until they're opaque. Toss them in a bowl with mixed greens, cherry

tomatoes, and grilled corn off the cob. Drizzle with a lemon-herb vinaigrette. This salad is a light and fresh testament to the sea's bounty.

Healthy Hand-Held Dinners

26. **Quinoa & Black Bean Burgers:** Combine cooked quinoa, mashed black beans, breadcrumbs, chopped cilantro, and a hint of cumin. Form into patties and grill until they sport a crispy crust. Serve these on whole wheat buns with avocado slices, lettuce, and a dab of Greek yogurt. A veggie burger that's hearty and packed with protein, it's a delightful change from the usual.

27. **Chicken & Veggie Fajitas:** Sauté thinly sliced chicken breast with bell peppers and onions, seasoned with chili and a touch of lime juice. Serve in whole wheat tortillas with a sprinkle of low-fat cheese and fresh pico de gallo. Roll it up, and every bite gives a zest of flavors and colors, making dinner vibrant and delicious.

28. **Stuffed Portobello Mushrooms:** Remove the stems from Portobello mushrooms and fill the caps with a mix of diced tomatoes, spinach, feta cheese, and Italian herbs. Grill until the mushrooms are tender and the cheese is slightly melted. Hold it by the cap and savor this juicy, earthy delight brimming with Mediterranean flavors.

29. **Spicy Lentil Tacos:** Sauté diced onions and garlic. Mix in cooked green lentils with spices: cumin, chili powder, and paprika. Load this mix into corn tortillas topped with diced tomatoes and lettuce. Add a sprinkle of queso fresco and a drizzle of lime-tinged Greek yogurt. A meatless, protein-packed dinner that's flavor-filled and health-conscious. Enjoy the spicy warmth in every bite!

29 HEALTHY SNACK IDEAS

1. **Crunchy Chickpeas:** Oven-roast chickpeas with olive oil, turmeric, and paprika.

2. **Greek Yogurt & Berries:** Mix fresh berries into plain Greek yogurt.

3. **Veggie Hummus Dip:** Slice carrots and cucumbers; dip into rich hummus.

4. **Almond Butter Celery:** Spread almond butter onto celery sticks.

5. **Quinoa Salad:** Toss cooked quinoa with diced veggies and lemon zest.

6. **Spiced Nuts:** Roast your favorite nuts with cayenne and honey.

7. **Avocado Toast:** Mashed avocado on whole grain toast. Sprinkle with sea salt.

8. **Cottage Cheese Bowl:** Mix cottage cheese with pineapple chunks.

9. **Chocolate-Dipped Strawberries:** Melt dark chocolate and dip strawberries.

10. **Edamame:** Steam and sprinkle with sea salt for a warm, protein-filled snack.

11. **Hard-Boiled Eggs:** Slice and sprinkle with salt and pepper.

12. **Chia Pudding:** Mix chia seeds in almond milk and refrigerate.

13. **Kale Chips:** Oven-bake kale with olive oil.

14. **Mixed Berries:** Fresh bowl of blueberries, raspberries, and blackberries.

15. **Sweet Potato Fries:** Oven-roast thin slices with olive oil.

16. **Apple Slices & Nut Butter:** Fresh apple slices paired with your favorite nut butter.

17. **Granola & Milk:** Crunchy granola immersed in cold almond milk.

18. **Tuna Salad:** Mix tuna, Greek yogurt, and dill.

19. **Cacao Nib Trail Mix:** Mix almonds, raisins, and cacao nibs.

20. **Fruit Leather:** Natural fruit purees dried into sweet sheets.

21. **Olive Medley:** Mix of green and black olives.

22. **Popcorn:** Air-pop and sprinkle with nutritional yeast.

23. **Protein Smoothie:** Blend spinach, protein powder, banana, strawberries, and almond milk.

24. **Roasted Seaweed:** Crispy sheets seasoned lightly.

25. **Frozen Grapes:** Freeze grapes for a chilled, sweet bite.

26. **Whole Wheat Crackers & Cheese:** Pair your favorite cheese with whole wheat crackers.

27. **Rice Cakes & Avocado:** Sliced avocado on rice cakes.

28. **Pistachios:** Shell and enjoy.

29. **Dried Apricots:** Chewy, sweet, and packed with nutrients.

KEEPING THE GAME ALIVE

Hey there, awesome reader! You've made it to the end, and now you're equipped with all the secrets to boost your health and energy with intermittent fasting. It's pretty exciting, right? But guess what? Your journey doesn't end here. It's time to share the magic and help others find their way too.

By sharing your thoughts about this book on Amazon, you're not just leaving a review. You're guiding other fantastic women over 50, just like you, to a place where they can discover how to feel their best every day. It's like passing on a secret recipe for health and happiness!

Your opinion is super valuable. It helps other ladies to find this book and learn all about feeling great and enjoying life to the fullest. And, by doing so, you're keeping the spirit of wellness and vibrant living alive and kicking!

So, could you take a tiny moment to leave your honest review? Every word you write helps more than you can imagine.

Thank you so much for your help. Together, we're keeping the joy of health and energy alive for women everywhere.

Simply scan the QR code below to leave your review:

And remember, each review is a step towards helping another wonderful woman find her path to a healthier, happier life. You're amazing for being part of this journey!

CONCLUSION

EMBRACING A F.A.S.T.W.I.S.E. FUTURE

As we wrap up our journey together, let's take a moment to reflect on the core message of this book: the F.A.S.T.W.I.S.E. system. Remember, this method isn't just a catchy acronym; it's a roadmap designed to make intermittent fasting simpler and more effective for you.

Throughout our time together, we've discussed the different elements of F.A.S.T.W.I.S.E., each carefully selected to address a specific aspect of your IF journey. From understanding the foundation of IF to setting tangible, actionable goals, every step along the way is crucial.

But here's what's truly special about F.A.S.T.W.I.S.E.: it's crafted with you, the incredible women over 50, in mind! I've spent years in the health and fitness field and seen firsthand how age can bring its share of unique challenges. That's why I've always felt that any health approach, especially something as powerful as IF, needs to be tailored to fit those unique needs. You are a beautiful, unique individual, and IF will work with you (not against you) to optimize your well-being.

Remember when we talked about setting achievable goals? It wasn't just about weight loss; it was about feeling empowered, rejuvenated, and strong in this phase of life. That's the beauty of the F.A.S.T.W.I.S.E. approach – it recognizes your individuality and embraces it wholeheartedly!

THE UNIQUE POWER OF IF FOR WOMEN OVER 50

Intermittent fasting isn't just another trend. It's here to stay and can make a huge difference in our lives, even as our bodies evolve. Our metabolism changes, menopause knocks on our doors, and we might notice weight creeping up in places it never used to. Through these transitions, IF can provide a great deal of help and some hope as well!

What's truly remarkable about IF is its adaptability. It's not about denying yourself or sticking to a rigid plan. It's about listening to your body and adjusting your eating patterns in a way that supports your personal journey. I remember when I first explored IF, I was amazed at how it allowed me to sync with my body's natural rhythms, especially during menopause.

The metabolic advantages of IF are undeniable. There is no doubt that our metabolism slows down over the years. Fortunately, IF can give it the boost it needs and can help our bodies burn off pesky fat more efficiently. Plus, if you take the hormonal benefits it can provide during menopause, you have yourself a secret weapon that can keep you feeling your absolute best.

Every woman's experience with IF will be personal. It's not about comparing yourself to others or striving for perfection. It's about understanding your body's needs, being patient with yourself, and embracing a journey that promises health, vitality, and empowerment, regardless of age.

Beyond Just Fasting

Intermittent fasting is more than just choosing when to eat; it's about creating a complete lifestyle change. From my own experience and countless stories shared with me, it's clear that diving headfirst into fasting without a clear mindset can lead to some uncomfortable hurdles.

Before starting, ask yourself, "Why am I choosing this path?" Having a clear purpose motivates us even on the most challenging days. When I began my IF journey, I took a weekend to really reflect on my goals. Was I looking for weight loss? Better health? Both? It's essential to know what you're aiming for, to measure your progress, and to celebrate your victories, no matter how small they may seem.

Then there's the physical aspect. While fasting can boost metabolism, pairing it with a balanced exercise routine maximizes its benefits. I found that even simple exercises, like daily walks or light stretching, significantly impacted how I felt and how much energy I had.

Of course, what you eat during your eating window also plays a massive role in your success. Nutritious, balanced meals ensure you get the most out of IF. Remember, it's not about eating less; it's about eating right.

Lastly, always appreciate the power of emotional well-being. Life can throw curveballs, and having a support system, be it friends, family, or an online community, can be a lifeline. Sharing your journey, both the highs and the lows, can make the path smoother and more enjoyable. Remember, holistic health isn't just about your body; it's also about your mind and spirit.

Your Health Odyssey Continues

One of the most inspiring stories I've heard is from a dear friend, Lisa. At 55, she found herself at a crossroads, realizing that the years were not just numbers but opportunities. Intermittent fasting wasn't her immediate go-to. In fact, she stumbled upon it while looking for a sustainable way to regain her energy and shed some unwanted weight that had crept on over the years. What started as an experiment soon became a routine, then a dedicated commitment.

But the transformation didn't happen overnight. Lisa faced challenges as she tried to adjust her eating windows and identify foods that sustained her energy. She read, researched, and noted how her body felt each day. It was this dedication to listening to her body that made all the difference. She learned that her journey with intermittent fasting was uniquely hers and that realization was empowering.

As her energy levels rose, Lisa rediscovered her love for the outdoors. What started as short, breathless walks turned into long, exhilarating hikes. She found herself waking up earlier, eager to hit the trails. Mountain hiking, something she never imagined attempting (even in her youth), became her life's passion. She shared how each summit she reached was a reminder of all of the barriers she had broken, both physically and mentally.

Her transformation went beyond the physical changes. Yes, she lost weight, but more importantly, she gained a new perspective on life. She spoke more confidently, tackled challenges head-on, and showed inspiring resilience. Lisa's journey reminds us that we're capable of incredible feats at any age. Her glowing spirit and healthy body were not just the results of intermittent fasting but her holistic approach to change. If there's anything to learn from her story, it's that commitment to yourself and your goals opens up endless possibilities, and it's never too late to redefine your life's journey.

Your journey with intermittent fasting doesn't end after the 29th day, nor does it conclude when you turn the last page of this book. It's an ongoing expedition, a commitment to yourself, where every day brings a new opportunity for growth, discovery, and vitality.

You're not alone on this path. Thousands of women, including myself, walk alongside you, each with their stories, insights, and endless wisdom. I urge you to join the broader community, share your experiences, and learn from one another. Together, we can uplift, inspire, and guide each other.

If you've found value in this guide, consider sharing it. Passing this book to a friend or family member is like giving the gift of health, an act of love that keeps on giving.

Lastly, your feedback is invaluable. Please take a moment to leave a review. Your insights help others on their journey and provide guidance for future editions. Remember, every step forward is a step towards a healthier you! I am so proud of you for taking this first step towards better health! By taking this bold first step, you are setting the stage for transformations far beyond what you can imagine right now. Today is a new chapter for you, and your hopes and dreams of better well-being await discovery. Keep going, keep pushing, and never give up. The best version of yourself is waiting to introduce herself!

REFERENCES

Intermittent Fasting: What is it, and how does it work? (2023, September 29). Johns Hopkins Medicine. https://www.hopkinsmedicine.org/health/wellness-and-prevention/intermittent-fasting-what-is-it-and-how-does-it-work

BSc, K. G. (2023, August 29). *Intermittent Fasting 101 — The Ultimate Beginner's Guide.* Healthline. https://www.healthline.com/nutrition/intermittent-fasting-guide

JustCook. (n.d.). *JustCook | FRESH MADE EASY.* https://justcook.ae/blog/intermittent-fasting-history-modern-adaptation-benefits

Schenkman, L. (2022, October 16). *The science behind intermittent fasting — and how you can make it work for you.* ideas.ted.com. https://ideas.ted.com/the-science-behind-intermittent-fasting-and-how-you-can-make-it-work-for-you/

Montgomery, M. (n.d.). *Is intermittent fasting the diet for you? Here's what the science says.* The Conversation. https://theconversation.com/is-intermittent-fasting-the-diet-for-you-heres-what-the-science-says-179454

Bauer, E. (2023, September 12). *Does Intermittent Fasting Work? A Science-Based Answer – KHNI.* Kerry Health and Nutrition Institute. https://khni.kerry.com/news/blog/does-intermittent-fasting-work-a-science-based-answer/

Research on intermittent fasting shows health benefits. (2020, February 27). National Institute on Aging. https://www.nia.nih.gov/news/research-intermittent-fasting-shows-health-benefits

Bauer, E. (2023c, September 12). *Does Intermittent Fasting Work? A Science-Based Answer – KHNI.* Kerry Health and Nutrition Institute. https://khni.kerry.com/news/blog/does-intermittent-fasting-work-a-science-based-answer/

Intermittent Fasting For Seniors: The Key To Staying Young & Living Longer - WeFast. (n.d.). https://www.wefast.care/articles/intermittent-fasting-for-seniors

What to know about intermittent fasting for women after 50. (2021, March 22). WebMD. https://www.webmd.com/healthy-aging/what-to-know-about-intermittent-fasting-for-women-after-50

Ruscio. (2023, September 19). What to Know About Intermittent Fasting For Women Over 50 - Dr. Michael Ruscio, DC. *Dr. Michael Ruscio, DC.* https://drruscio.com/fasting-for-women-over-50/

Anton, S. D., Ezzati, A., Witt, D., McLaren, C., & Vial, P. (2021). The effects of intermittent fasting regimens in middle-age and older adults: Current state of evidence. *Experimental Gerontology, 156,* 111617. https://doi.org/10.1016/j.exger.2021.111617

Domaszewski, P., Konieczny, M., Pakosz, P., Łukaniszyn-Domaszewska, K., Mikuláková, W., Sadowska-Krępa, E., & Anton, S. (2022). Effect of a six-week times restricted eating intervention on the body composition in early elderly men with overweight. *Scientific Reports, 12*(1). https://doi.org/10.1038/s41598-022-13904-9

Vasim, I., Majeed, C. N., & DeBoer, M. D. (2022b). Intermittent fasting and metabolic health. *Nutrients, 14*(3), 631. https://doi.org/10.3390/nu14030631

Nazish, N. (2021, June 30). 10 Intermittent fasting myths You should Stop believing. *Forbes.* https://www.forbes.com/sites/nomanazish/2021/06/30/10-intermittent-fasting-myths-you-should-stop-believing/?sh=660e0177335b

Stanton, B. (2020). 7 Common intermittent fasting myths, debunked. *HUM Nutrition Blog.* https://www.humnutrition.com/blog/intermittent-fasting-myths/

Stone, D. (2017). A Beginners guide to intermittent fasting. *Dawna Stone.* https://dawnastone.com/wp-content/uploads/2017/11/Intermittent-Fasting-Checklist.pdf

Recovery, L. (2023, June 13). *Understanding Detox: What is Medically Supervised Withdrawal?* Landmark Recovery. https://landmarkrecovery.com/understanding-detox/

Detoxification: A Natural Bonus Of Intermittent Fasting - WeFast. (n.d.). https://www.wefast.care/articles/detoxification-a-natural-bonus-of-intermittent-fasting#:

Soler, R. (2021). Intermittent Fasting: Does it help detox your body? *SparnDetox.* https://sparndetox.com/blogs/news/intermittent-fasting-does-it-help-detox-your-body

Cornish, R. (2021, November 10). The Fasting Fix - How to Detoxify Successfully and Stay Nourished. • Move Nourish Change. *Move Nourish Change.* https://movenourishchange.com/2021/11/04/the-fasting-fix-how-to-detoxify-successfully-and-stay-nourished/

Lutsiv, N., & Fleming, K. (2023). Fasting Detox: Foods And Drinks To Detoxify Your Body Safely. *BetterMe Blog.* https://betterme.world/articles/fasting-detox/

Hahn-Chaney, R. (2022). #168 - Don't Break The 12-Hour Gap: Health Tips for Intermittent Fasting — Run To The Best You. *Run to the Best You.* https://www.runtothebestyou.com/news-notes/don%E2%80%99t-break-the-12-hour-gap-health-tips-for-intermittent-fasting#:

Fasting & Detox Coaching comprehensive guide | Bodhi Holistic Hub. (n.d.). https://www.bodhiholistichub.com/learning-hub/holistic-modality-guides/natural-medicine/fasting-detox-coaching

Swaine, A. (2020). Intermittent fasting as a detox tool — FASTING+. *FASTING+.* https://nutritionistsblend.com/blog/blog-post-title-one-xxkry

"Detoxes" and "Cleanses": What You Need To Know. (n.d.). NCCIH. https://www.nccih.nih.gov/health/detoxes-and-cleanses-what-you-need-to-know

Detoxification to Promote Health: A Seven Day Program. (n.d.). University of Wisconsin School of Medicine and Health. https://www.fammed.wisc.edu/files/webfm-uploads/documents/outreach/im/handout_detoxplan.pdf

Leonard, J. (2023, March 6). *Six ways to do intermittent fasting*. https://www.medicalnewstoday.com/articles/322293

Canning, K., & Talbert, S. (2022, October 3). 6 Popular Intermittent Fasting Schedules For Weight Loss, Explained By Experts. *Women's Health*. https://www.womenshealthmag.com/weight-loss/a29349587/intermittent-fasting-schedule/

Migala, J. (2022, March 11). *7 types of intermittent fasting: Which is best for you?* EverydayHealth.com. https://www.everydayhealth.com/diet-nutrition/diet/types-intermittent-fasting-which-best-you/

Finding Your Unique & Optimal Fasting Window. (n.d.). Lumen. Retrieved October 21, 2023, from https://www.lumen.me/blog/nutrition/find-out-which-intermittent-fasting-schedule-will-work-for-you

Cohen, M. (2023, February 6). 10 best intermittent fasting apps for weight loss. *Good Housekeeping*. https://www.goodhousekeeping.com/health-products/g34618367/best-apps-intermittent-fasting/

How to create an intermittent fasting schedule - FreshCap Mushrooms. (2020, December 4). FreshCap Mushrooms. https://learn.freshcap.com/tips/how-to-create-an-intermittent-fasting-schedule/

Eenfeldt, A. (2022, November 4). *Intermittent fasting success stories - Diet Doctor*. Diet Doctor. https://www.dietdoctor.com/intermittent-fasting/success-stories

Wilslm. (n.d.). *Reddit - Dive into anything*. https://www.reddit.com/r/intermittentfasting/comments/v6z92j/any_success_stories_for_40_women/

Snow_Soldier. (n.d.-b). *Reddit - Dive into anything*. https://www.reddit.com/r/xxfitness/comments/658oti/intermittent_fasting_success_stories

Fasting: How to prepare your mind, body, and fasting tools. (2022, April 15). Redmond Life. https://redmond.life/blogs/live-your-journey/fasting-how-to-prepare-your-mind-body-and-fasting-tools

Miller, K. (2022). 8 tips to start intermittent fasting and stick with it. *Women's Health*. https://www.womenshealthmag.com/weight-loss/a38191815/starting-sticking-with-intermittent-fasting/

C. (2020). How To Prepare Yourself Before Starting Intermittent Fasting. *Meds News – Health and Medicine Information*. https://www.medsnews.com/health/preparing-before-intermittent-fasting/

What are the rules of intermittent fasting? (2021, December 30). https://www.hackensackmeridianhealth.org/en/healthu/2021/12/30/what-are-the-rules-of-intermittent-fasting

Rd, R. a. M. (2023, July 31). *What are the different stages of fasting?* Healthline. https://www.healthline.com/nutrition/stages-of-fasting#:

Intermittent fasting may help these 7 common medical conditions. (2023, March 2). Rupa Health. https://www.rupahealth.com/post/7-medical-conditions-that-intermittent-fasting-can-help

Buckingham, C., & Buckingham, C. (2022). 11 people who should never try intermittent fasting. *Eat This Not That.* https://www.eatthis.com/is-intermit tent-fasting-safe/

Intermittent fasting - setting solid goals for success. (n.d.). https://www.peakperfor mancehabits.com/blog/intermittent-fasting-setting-goals-success

Fletcher, J. (2023, January 5). *How to begin intermittent fasting.* https://www.medicalnewstoday.com/articles/324882

Colbert, K., & Colbert, K. (2023). Setting your IF Goals and Expectations: A guide to successful Intermittent fasting. *Intermittent Fasting 16/8.* https://if168.com/blogs/if-16-8-challenge/setting-your-if-goals-and-expectations-a-guide-to-successful-intermittent-fasting

DaedricDweller. (n.d.). *Reddit - Dive into anything.* https://www.reddit.com/r/intermittentfasting/comments/ry1s3v/best_plan_or_time_to_set_as_a_goal/

Akadaedalus. (n.d.). *Reddit - Dive into anything.* https://www.reddit.com/r/intermittentfasting/comments/md1z08/setting_goals_how_much_is_too_much/

Rd, N. G. (2023). How to Prepare for fasting: An In-Depth Guide. *Zero Longevity.* https://zerolongevity.com/blog/preparing-for-a-fast/

Top 10 intermittent fasting tips that will help you stay on track – Align Brooklyn. (n.d.). https://alignbrooklyn.com/top-10-intermittent-fasting-tips-that-will-help-you-stay-on-track/

Miller, K. (2022b). 8 tips to start intermittent fasting and stick with it. *Women's Health.* https://www.womenshealthmag.com/weight-loss/a38191815/starting-sticking-with-intermittent-fasting/

Medical Device News Magazine & Medical Device News Magazine, a division of PTM Healthcare Marketing, Inc. (2021, December 10). Intermittent Fasting - Diet Tips To Stay On Track - Medical Device News Magazine. *Medical Device News Magazine.* https://infomeddnews.com/intermittent-fasting-diet-tips-to-stay-on-track/

Cpt, A. B. C. M. B. (2021, July 16). 10 Best Liquids To Drink While Fasting For Fat Loss. *AutumnElleNutrition.* https://www.autumnellenutrition.com/post/10-best-liquids-to-drink-while-fasting-for-fat-loss

Best And Worst Intermittent Fasting Drinks. (2022, July 4). FUL. https://fulcompany.com/blogs/the-ful-scoop/drinks-for-intermittent-fasting

Meier, M. (2021, September 8). What snacks can you eat when you're intermittent fasting? *Bodyandsoul*. https://www.bodyandsoul.com.au/nutrition/what-snacks-can-you-eat-when-youre-intermittent-fasting/news-story/88caffe34b9f62a1f619d3b1f8ca5581

Rizzo, N. (2020). What foods are best to eat on an intermittent fasting diet? *Greatist*. https://greatist.com/eat/what-to-eat-on-an-intermittent-fasting-diet

Chien, S., Howley, E. K., & Burdeos, J. (2023, September 8). What is intermittent fasting? *US News & World Report*. https://health.usnews.com/wellness/food/articles/intermittent-fasting-foods-to-eat-and-avoid

Shinners, R., & Berry, E. (2022, November 21). 101 short exercise quotes to keep you motivated and inspired. *Woman's Day*. https://www.womansday.com/health-fitness/g2318/healthy-lifestyle-quotes/

Lindberg, S. (2023, May 4). *How to exercise safely during intermittent fasting*. Healthline. https://www.healthline.com/health/how-to-exercise-safely-intermittent-fasting

Working Out While Intermittent Fasting. (n.d.). Prospect Medical Systems. Retrieved October 21, 2023, from https://www.prospectmedical.com/resources/wellness-center/working-out-while-intermittent-fasting

CSCS, A. H., & Ritchey, C. (2023, September 22). What to know about intermittent fasting and your workouts. *Men's Health*. https://www.menshealth.com/fitness/a30300614/intermittent-fasting-working-out/

Kamb, S., & Kamb, S. (2023). How To Build Your Own Workout Routine (Plans & Exercises). *Nerd Fitness*. https://www.nerdfitness.com/blog/how-to-build-your-own-workout-routine/

Fitness program: 5 steps to get started. (2021, December 16). Mayo Clinic. https://www.mayoclinic.org/healthy-lifestyle/fitness/in-depth/fitness/art-20048269

Grmn. (n.d.). *Reddit - Dive into anything*. https://www.reddit.com/r/productivity/comments/116lli5/how_to_combine_intermittent_fasting_waking_up/

Gooner. (n.d.). *Reddit - Dive into anything*. https://www.reddit.com/r/intermittentfasting/comments/urnz78/people_who_do_168_fast_when_do_you_workout/

DrGarciaIdaho. (2020, June 5). *Struggling with Intermittent Fasting? - Idaho Center for Functional Medicine*. Idaho Center for Functional Medicine. https://www.drpaulgarciadc.com/struggling-with-intermittent-fasting/

BodyFast App, We ♥ fasting, Lose weight the healthy way, without a diet. (2017). The surprising link between intermittent fasting and allergies. *BodyFast App | We ♥ Fasting | Lose Weight the Healthy Way, Without a Diet | Lose Weight, Feel Great and Get Fit*. https://www.bodyfast.app/en/fasting-reduces-allergic-reactions/#:

4 Intermittent Fasting Side Effects to Watch Out For. (n.d.). Harvad Health

Publishing. Retrieved October 21, 2023, from https://www.health.harvard. edu/staying-healthy/4-intermittent-fasting-side-effects-to-watch-out-for https://www.mynetdiary.com/what-to-eat-during-intermittent-fasting.html

Minus, D. P. (2023, May 19). Intermittent fasting and social eating: How to handle dining out and family gatherings. *Diet Plus Minus*. https://www.diet plusminus.com/post/intermittent-fasting-and-social-eating-how-to-handle-dining-out-and-family-gatherings

Dieker, N. (2020, February 23). *Does intermittent fasting work for moms?* Blog | Haven Life. https://havenlife.com/blog/intermittent-fasting-moms/

BodyFast App, We 🖤 fasting, Lose weight the healthy way, without a diet. (2021). 5 Ways to Stay Motivated when Doing Intermittent Fasting. *BodyFast App | We 🖤 Fasting | Lose Weight the Healthy Way, Without a Diet | Lose Weight, Feel Great and Get Fit*. https://www.bodyfast.app/en/motivation-for-intermit tent-fasting/

Geurin, L. (2023). 7 Ways to Stay Motivated when fasting: Tips for intermittent fasting success. *LoriGeurin.com | Wellness for Life*. https://lorigeurin.com/fast ing-motivation/

Rd, K. M. (2023). 8 Powerful ways to find encouragement + motivation for fast-ing. *Zero Longevity*. https://zerolongevity.com/blog/motivation-for-fasting/

Sugar, J. (2020, May 26). How I stay Motivated to do intermittent fasting | POPSUGAR Fitness. *POPSUGAR Fitness*. https://www.popsugar.com/ fitness/how-i-stay-motivated-to-do-intermittent-fasting-47460042

Anarkyfilms. (n.d.). *Reddit - Dive into anything*. https://www.reddit.com/r/inter mittentfasting/comments/qheur2/how_to_stay_motivated/

Menopause - Symptoms and causes - Mayo Clinic. (2023, May 25). Mayo Clinic. https://www.mayoclinic.org/diseases-conditions/menopause/symptoms-causes/syc-20353397

Admin-Midday. (2023, August 21). *Menopause and intermittent fasting - Plus 5 tips for doing it right - Midday*. Midday. https://midday.health/blog/menopause-and-intermittent-fasting-plus-5-tips-for-doing-it-right/

Seo, R. D. (n.d.). » *Intermittent fasting during menopause: What do you need to know?* https://www.menopausecentre.com.au/information-centre/articles/inter mittent-fasting-during-menopause-what-do-you-need-to-know/

Cpt, K. D. M. R. (2021, September 20). *The definitive guide to healthy eating in your 50s and 60s*. Healthline. https://www.healthline.com/nutrition/healthy-eating-50s-60s

Carter, C. (2023). What should your diet be like after 50? *AARP*. https://www. aarp.org/health/healthy-living/info-2020/nutrition-after-age-50.html

Chen, L. (2019). The best diet for women over 50. *LIVESTRONG.COM*. https:// www.livestrong.com/article/443814-balanced-diet-for-a-50-year-old-female/

National Academies Press (US). (2004). *Weight-Loss and maintenance strategies.* Weight Management - NCBI Bookshelf. https://www.ncbi.nlm.nih.gov/books/NBK221839/

Scripps Health. (2023, May 23). How to support someone on their weight loss journey. *Scripps Health.* https://www.scripps.org/news_items/7603-how-to-support-someone-on-their-weight-loss-journey

Bouchez, C. (2006, February 10). *10 ways to help a loved one lose weight.* WebMD. https://www.webmd.com/obesity/features/10-ways-to-help-a-loved-one-lose-weight

Cpt, A. B. C. M. B. (2022, August 15). 5 Intermittent Fasting Break-Fast Recipes For EVERY Situation! (Traveling, Brunch, At Work). *AutumnElleNutrition.* https://www.autumnellenutrition.com/post/5-intermittent-fasting-break-fast-recipes-for-every-situation-traveling-brunch-at-work

Intermittent fasting breakfast recipes. (n.d.). Pinterest. https://www.pinterest.com/autumnellenutrition/intermittent-fasting-breakfast-recipes/

the Daily Connoisseur. (2022, February 17). *Intermittent Fasting Teas + 10 breakfast Ideas* [Video]. YouTube. https://www.youtube.com/watch?v=44nAtK1l7qo

Ganguly, R. (2023, May 25). *On intermittent fasting diet? try these breakfast options.* Slurrp. https://www.slurrp.com/article/on-intermittent-fasting-diet-try-these-breakfast-options-1684984055691

32 top intermittent fasting recipes - Food.com. (2020, March 2). https://www.food.com/ideas/intermittent-fasting-recipes-6939

5:2 diet recipes | BBC Good Food. (2022, November 24). https://www.bbcgoodfood.com/recipes/collection/5-2-recipes

Apd, L. B. R. (2023). 16/8 intermittent fasting 7-day meal plan for beginners. *Simple.life Blog.* https://simple.life/blog/16-8-intermittent-fasting-7-day-meal-plan/

www.weightlossresources.co.uk. (n.d.). *5:2 Diet recipes: 34 easy meals under 300 calories.* https://www.weightlossresources.co.uk/recipes/5-2-diet-fasting-day.htm

BodyFast App, We 🧡 fasting, Lose weight the healthy way, without a diet. (2021b). Top Snacks for Successful Weight Loss with Fasting. *BodyFast App | We 🧡 Fasting | Lose Weight the Healthy Way, Without a Diet | Lose Weight, Feel Great and Get Fit.* https://www.bodyfast.app/en/healthy-snacks/

Munuhe, N., & Fleming, K. (2023). Intermittent Fasting Snacks: 10 Plus Healthy Bitings That Will Help You Stay On Track. *BetterMe Blog.* https://betterme.world/articles/intermittent-fasting-snacks/

Mba, A. L. B. (2023, May 4). *29 Healthy snacks that can help you lose weight.* Healthline. https://www.healthline.com/nutrition/29-healthy-snacks-for-weight-loss#TOC_TITLE_HDR_4

Ryan. (2023). Intermittent fasting meal plan. *Ryan and Alex*. https://www.ryanandalex.com/intermittent-fasting-meal-plan/

Abstract Doodle Brown Meal Planner. (2022, March 17). https://wepik.com/template/simple-weekly-diet-meal-planner-r-1655457637

Printed in Great Britain
by Amazon

38193816R00106